Heartbeat:
The Politics of Health Research

Heartbeat:
The Politics of Health Research

Natalie Davis Spingarn

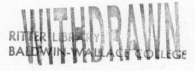
Robert B. Luce, Inc.   Washington-New York

Spingarn, Natalie Davis.
    Heartbeat: the politics of health research.

    Includes bibliographical references and index.
    1. United States. National Institutes of
Health. 2. Medical research—United States.
I. Title.
RA11. D6S63   353.008'41   75-28551
ISBN 0-88331-081-3

Contents

For My Parents

Introduction

Turn on the television, pick up a magazine, and you have evidence of our fascination with medical discoveries which promise relief from pain, or longer life. Considering this fascination, it has always seemed strange to me that so few outside the world of medical science recognize the name of the government's chief agency for effecting these discoveries or know about the policy issues which eddy around it.

This is a book about that agency, the National Institutes of Health (NIH). It is a book about the biomedical scientists, administrators and others who work at the agency's Bethesda headquarters and in NIH-supported research around the country (who, together with their alumni-advocates, I have called "the NIHers"). It is a book about their relationship with the government of which NIH is an unusual part, and how this relationship has influenced the scientists' search for knowledge about our health.

It is a book, then, about the politics of health research. Webster's says politics is, "the art or science concerned with guiding or influencing policy". This is not an angry book, neither is it a panegyric. It tries to cast light rather than heat on the issues that have developed over the past 30 years as American politics has made possible the development of a $2 billion-a-year health research effort which has played a major role in revolutionizing the practice of medicine.

At the moment, the National Institutes of Health stands at

a crossroads. It cannot go back to its early years, when a Congress generous in bestowing funds tiptoed lightly so as not to disturb genius at work. It cannot stand still. It has been through some difficult years, in which elected and appointed officials have tried to hurry, direct and divide its work, and not always tactfully. Now it must enter a new era in which it continues to foster the search for knowledge while finding an accommodation with modern public demands.

Whether or not NIH succeeds depends in good measure on general understanding of the policy questions involved. All patients and future patients have a stake in the outcome. Yet little has been written about these issues outside the specialized literature. Hence this attempt to elucidate them for a wider readership.

Immense government institutions are difficult to penetrate; behind great walls, they speak their own languages and pursue their own folkways. I have chosen to look at NIH by examining one of its eleven Institutes through a microscope rather than to look at all of them through a panoramic lens. The National Heart and Lung Institute (NHLI) is not a typical institute. None is. But it resembles the others closely, and it deals with dramatic major disease problems affecting us all; its people, projects, history, successes, frustrations and current problems can serve as a good case in point. Through the vignettes at the beginning of each chapter, I have tried to personify the issues with which that chapter deals and so relate technical material to individual lives.

We open with a brief chapter on the Institutes today, then step backwards to the Golden Years which saw the blossoming of the great health research effort centered in Bethesda, and the foreboding criticism that developed as those years drew to a close. How to reap more health research results more quickly and in such a way that they are most helpful to more patients? We explore that central issue in the next chapters: chapter three on the individual investigators who initiate their own projects and the challenge to that approach during the War on

2

Cancer; chapter four on the newer approach to health research mandated by a Congress seeking more relevance and "accountability" (as seen in microcosm at Dr. Michael DeBakey's Heart and Blood Vessel Supercenter in Houston). And in the Disease of the Month Club chapter, we deal with the increased, more scattered directives to NIH from the public and its representatives, and one highly talented NHLI investigator's reaction to them.

All such forces affect an Institute's program. In the sixth chapter, we look at the NHLI's overall program across the continuum from basic research through clinical trials to demonstration and education programs which seek to control disease. Here we will see how one Institute spends the funds the Congress allots as a result of the long political process; the choices which budget limitations impose on even this favored institute, and the resulting squeeze on the traditional individual or "basic" investigator.

Chapters seven and eight explore topics vital to the continued operation of health research. Research training is a complex, confused topic, but it is crucial to the future of the whole system. The Totally Implantable Artificial Heart story raises questions about the relationship of medical research to the entire society—how the fruits of its work should be distributed and paid for, and, indeed, whether some should be developed at all. The final chapter summarizes today's pressures and their effects on the NIHers and their work.

Researching the researchers has not been an easy job. Traditionally, the NIHers have been protected from public scrutiny. There is a culture gap, too. Some in the ranks are caught short even by the word "politics," which has x-rated connotations and is still often thought of as the small shrewd ways people deal with each other in organizations rather than its true sense. I have covered the NIHers for many years. As a government official in the Department of Health, Education, and Welfare and on Capitol Hill, I have worked with them. Now I find, happily, that many of them are becoming more conscious of the need to explain what they are doing to the public.

I taped some 75 interviews in the course of writing this book, at Bethesda, on Capitol Hill, in downtown Washington, and at facilities around the country. I attended many committee meetings on NIH concerns, including National Heart and Lung Advisory Council sessions, Congressional hearings and the President's Biomedical Research Panel meetings. The Panel's hearings proved a bonanza, not only since they brought together the whole panoply of figures associated with health research and its problems, but also because under the Freedom of Information Act, I had access to the many helpful documents prepared by the staff or submitted by outside witnesses.

A few reservations: events move swiftly in political Washington; what is considered to be fact one day may be outdated the next. Even the name of the National Heart and Lung Institute will probably have been changed (to include the word "Blood") by the time this book is published, and of course the Biomedical Research Panel will have finished its work and congressional committees will have held hearings on its recommendations. Knowing this, I have tried to focus on the general issues that will be with us for many years, no matter where the mantle of power may fall, or what the tinkering with institutional forms. I have had, of course, to write about the people who were on the scene in 1975 and 1976. Except where otherwise noted, my budget figures are for the fiscal year 1976 (July 1, 1975 - June 30, 1976, and even that format will change in the fall of 1976). And, unfortunately, I could not include all the material gathered; I had to be selective and try to concentrate on those people and events I thought best exemplified the issues.

It would be impossible for me to list all the people who have been helpful. First there were Dr. Theodore Cooper and the other principals whose names you will read, who submitted to long taped interviews, some as often as three or four times.

4

At NIH, the central Communications office, headed by Storm Whaley, opened many doors. My special thanks go to capable Irving Goldberg, who has an inexhaustible store of knowledge about the whole Public Health Service, and also to his aide, Nancy Coffin. G. Raymond Womeldorf, Jr. and his legislative staff were gracious in checking facts and figures. I am grateful to the NHLI's Director, Dr. Robert I. Levy and his staff, especially Dr. Jim L. Shields, Dr. Jerome Green, Dr. Donald MacCanon and Ernest Miner for their patience with my questioning and their responsiveness.

On Capitol Hill, I am indebted especially to Dr. David Banta, one of the new group of medical school faculty members first brought to Washington as a Robert Wood Johnson Health Policy Fellow. An internist and public health specialist with some cardiological training, and now a Hill staffer, he shared with me a draft study of NIH done for Congressman Paul Rogers' health subcommittee. Another NIH interview report by Dr. Jarold Kieffer of the President's Biomedical Research Panel staff also expanded my vantage point.

The whole Panel staff, especially Dr. George Eaves, was tolerant of my intrusions on their time, as were John Blamphin and Jane Fullarton of HEW's "H" office. Former NIH Deputy Director Dr. John Sherman, now at the Association of American Medical Colleges, was always ready to help in any way he could, providing information about the agency for which he holds such deep affection. These people and many others provided a wide diversity of views on many important matters; some reviewed the manuscript in part, or as a whole.

For skillful secretarial assistance I am grateful to Kathyrn Baker and to Paula Colozzi, who also assisted in reading proofs and offered many useful comments. Most of all, my thanks go to my husband, Jerome H. Spingarn, whose wise counsel, criticism and patience sustained me throughout.

The final product is mine, and I accept full responsibility for it. I hope that in its own small way, it will add to public understanding of the politics of health research, and thus enable this research to play an ever stronger role in improving our lives.

Natalie Davis Spingarn

March, 1976

1.   The Jewel That Lost Its Lustre

The Director's office in Building One has changed since Dr. Donald S. Fredrickson has taken over at the National Institutes of Health: Persian rugs grace both floor and tables, venerable Dutch furniture and prints—all from his own collection—have replaced Early Bureaucratic, and at the Building entrance, red carpeting has been laid. The third NIH Director of the Nixon-Ford Administrations is establishing his own image, his own leadership. He wears his white doctor's coat to staff meetings, reminding subordinates that he is a distinguished medical researcher, award winner and teacher as well as an administrator.

Some speak of his reserve and of the dignified formality he and his Dutch-born wife display. She is an attorney and businesswoman who sometimes presides as hostess at office luncheons served on her own delicate china. Others admire Fredrickson's charm and brilliance and the articulate, elegant prose in which he argues for such generalities as a restoration of "class" to the Institutes or for such specifics as a bridging of the "translation gap" between laboratory bench and bedside. An aide wonders whether Don Fredrickson, a Renaissance man himself— skier and pianist ("I'm working my way through 'The Well-Tempered Clavier'"), as well as scientist—can reestablish a Renaissance at the NIH and at the same time lead an agency which accepts its place in the ranks in the modern wars against disease.

Downtown, it's not so easy to make an impact. In the Senate Caucus Room beneath the ornate crystal chandeliers made world-famous during Watergate, Dr. Fredrickson joins a group of Department of Health, Education, and Welfare men testifying before Health Subcommittee Chairman Senator Edward M. Kennedy (who, months before, told a Harvard School of Public Health audience that those days in which NIH had been "a sacred cow" had passed). Assistant Secretary for Health Theodore Cooper reads the Administration position (negative) on the bill at hand. Though this measure aims to organize NIH better to deal with genetic diseases, and though NIH Director Fredrickson has co-edited the standard text "The Metabolic Basis of Inherited Disease", he gets to say very little. He is only part of a management-minded Administration team. Senator Kennedy appears bored; he cuts the hearing short; no real issues have been aired.

After the cold, arrogant hand of the Nixon Administration had lifted, the National Institutes of Health, central to the nation's health research effort, lay waiting. The chill winds of fall, then winter, cut across the rolling "campus" ten miles north of Washington, blowing against the busy 14 story Clinical Center with its some 500 hospital beds and 1,100 disease-studying laboratories, blowing against the academic brick and newer concrete and glass office buildings. The winds, both physical and political, often blew sharply. But they could not dispel the mood that touched the place and its 10,000 workers.

"Malaise," Dr. Donald Fredrickson described it, during his year of self-imposed exile at the National Academy of Sciences' Institute of Medicine downtown. And then, perhaps because he once headed the Heart Institute, and thinks in cardiological terms, he added "malaise de coeur".

Spring came. An enormous red and yellow striped awning was raised at the back of the campus to shelter the nearly 800 medical scientists attending the First NIH Alumni Reunion.

There were no beenies, no beer and pretzels under this tent, just rows of folding chairs and, along the walls, dry scientific exhibits depicting for the returning "alumni" the current work of the eleven Institutes.

Alumnus Dr. Arthur Kornberg, a Nobel Laureate from Stanford, set the tone. He said that the reunion had been convened not only to recall the past and present achievements of the Institutes, but to express concern for their future. Had our nation the good sense to develop national institutes of comparable status in agriculture and energy resources, many of our present problems would be less serious. Despite this, and despite the achievements of NIH, many of them of "stellar magnitude", the agency was being subjected to severe criticism. Its enlarged budget is now a vulnerable target for budget cutters and "antiscience" forces. Stand fast; as with all worthwhile things, the struggle for survival is never won. This is even more true for support of science than for other institutions in society.

Secretary of Health, Education, and Welfare Caspar Weinberger, "Cap the Knife", he of the sharp mind and even sharper budget cuts, rose next. He had, it was announced, brought the Reunion a present. Two former directors of the National Heart and Lung Institute, Doctors Donald S. Fredrickson and Theodore Cooper, would assume health leadership in the Ford-Rockefeller Administration: Fredrickson would direct NIH; Dr. Cooper would head "H", as the Republicans had dubbed the Public Health Service, or the six-agency health empire within HEW. (The bureaucratic mould changes frequently. As of this writing, H is made up of the Alcohol, Drug Abuse, and Mental Health Administration; the Center for Disease Control; the Food and Drug Administration; the Health Resources Administration and the Health Services Administration as well as the NIH.)

Enthusiastic applause greeted this announcement, signaling the relief the audience felt at having friends, NIH stalwarts both, in court. But would it make a difference? Could détente be established between NIH and its bioscientist-constituency

9

and those Arthur Kornberg had labeled the anti-scientists downtown? And what difference does it make anyway to the patient in pain out there with cancer, or heart disease, or diabetes?

To the casual observer passing through, NIH does not seem an orphaned child, a target for budget cutters and anti-scientists. On the contrary, NIH has a sleek and healthy, though in some spots, middle-aged, look. The government's health research agency is headquartered on 306 acres of verdant land, adorned with willows, maples, a stream, and carefully kept lawns. Ten of the Institutes have offices here: Aging; Allergy and Infectious Diseases; Arthritis, Metabolism, and Digestive Diseases; Cancer; Child Health and Human Development; Dental Research; Eye; General Medical Sciences; Heart and Lung; and Neurological and Communicative Disorders and Stroke. The eleventh—Environmental Health Sciences, which deals with a comparatively new human problem, the relationship between health and the environment—has begun its work at the Research Triangle Park in North Carolina.

Some say NIH resembles a favored university; after all, does it not have a serene aloof academic look, complete with on-campus houses for V.I.P.s like those of college presidents? And is that not a huge schematic cell on the front lawn in front of white columned Building One, put there for the Alumni Reunion—white, with multicolored trim and mirrored nucleus, its inner surfaces covered with phrases like *endoplasmic reticulum* or *Golgi apparatus*? What else could this be, except a university?

Others feel NIH more like a sprawling town, with its own library, hospital, apartment house, credit union, fire department, education and civil defense programs, telephone book and parking problems. If this be so, the central portion, like that of other towns, has room for most, but not all of the some 51 buildings which house animals and animal feed as well as working people; the others spill over into neighboring

10

Maryland suburbs; there is even an animal farm in exurban Poolesville. And of course, the population is most highly educated—2,280 professionals with doctorate degrees work here, almost equally divided into M.D.s and Ph.Ds (ten percent of the M.D.s have Ph.Ds as well) with dentists and veterinarians to round out the picture.

All this government brain power needs support, and gets it: people from other countries can scarcely believe their eyes and ears. Jean-Marie Matthieu, for one, a Swiss pediatrician who recently spent two years as a visiting scientist at the Neurological Institute describes the facilities in glowing terms in the May 10-11, 1975, weekend edition of *Neue Zurcher Zeitung*: the laboratories each with its own computerized budget ("whereby the balance can be obtained immediately"); the self-service supermarket where laboratory glassware, office supplies and instruments can be purchased with a credit card; the graphics department "which can produce anything conceivable in the audio-visual area"; the experimental animals ordered by telephone and delivered the same day. Besides the 100 mouse and rat strains, available in all age classes, NIH also has a monkey colony, cows, horses, germ-free animals and rare mutants.

As if this were not enough, Dr. Matthieu, a student of the human brain, reports on another feature of NIH he considers most unusual: the "total readiness to cooperate encountered on every level". No director or Nobel Prize winner would ever refuse to discuss a problem, he writes, there are no internal barriers, no scientific hierarchies: "One simply speaks to the person with the knowledge. Nobody at NIH would ever monopolize his equipment." It is possible to wander into a laboratory and use the tabletop calculators, centrifuges, scintillation counters, etc. Matthieu continues. In view of the high concentration of researchers in every area of medicine and biology, it is practically possible to find a respected specialist in every biomedical area within minutes, and these specialists are quite ready to provide information in their fields. It is also "extremely simple" to organize interdisciplinary projects, since all staff members are happy to participate in new projects if they are truly interesting.

The tall, red brick Clinical Center, site of much of the on-campus laboratory research Dr. Matthieu describes (known in bureaucratese as the NIH intramural effort) seems the busiest place at NIH, as well as the one in which Dr. Marcus Welby and his scriptwriters would be most at home. Like any major medical center nowadays, its halls and elevators are crowded with white coated doctors, nurses and armies of technicians and other aides. But unlike most such centers, though this is a hospital with over 500 beds and ambulatory care clinics, twice as much space is devoted to laboratories as to patient areas. Patients come from every corner of the United States, not because they choose this hospital, but because they suffer from an assortment of human ills under study here, from cancer to schizophrenia to epilepsy or muscular dystrophy. They are participants in research projects, as are the normal volunteers, largely young people from universities and church organizations, who provide the information about healthy people needed for comparison.

Such patients and volunteers have participated in a great deal of landmark research—in the search for a combination of drugs used effectively to treat patients with advanced Hodgkin's Disease, a cancer of the lymph system which was once usually fatal; in the finding which helped scientists understand the way the body rejects foreign substances; and in discovering the virus that causes one kind of hepatitis. But for most cure-hungry Americans, the Clinical Center may be less consequential than some of the more traditional office buildings where the Institutes' administrative and especially extramural staff is quartered, on and off the campus.

The intramural program is a model; in fact, it appears to be the single most productive biomedical research institution in the United States (in terms of articles published and influence per article). But the extramural program is where the money is. Only about ten percent of the $2 billion NIH budget is spent on intramural research; 70-80 percent goes through grants and contracts into research done elsewhere.

So NIH is not simply what you see in Bethesda, Maryland. The government's health research arm stretches far, far out to grantees and contractors largely in university medical centers and private laboratories in every state, and to some abroad. It has developed a complex series of relationships with these biomedical researchers and their colleagues different from those of any other government agency. Many of them trained in its intramural laboratories. Many serve on its peer review committees which evaluate and rate grant applications, or on its various advisory councils and committees. Its constituency has become a formidable one. Together with the central NIH staff, we may call them the "NIHers".

This then, is the government agency which President Lyndon B. Johnson's Secretary for Health, Education, and Welfare Wilbur J. Cohen called "the most precious jewel in the crown of H.E.W." Some say that in the early 1970s, that jewel lost some of its lustre. Surely morale fell as the agency became subject to political buffeting. Two directors were fired in less than two years. Discouraged, and in some cases, disgusted, a score of the top NIH leaders left for greener pastures, including two eminent deputy directors—Dr. Robert Berliner to become dean of Yale Medical School and Dr. John Sherman to be number two man at the Association of American Medical Colleges.

The experts say lustre can be restored to a jewel—its inner beauty brought out—if it is properly treated. In those early Nixon days that prospect seemed dim to NIHers both on and off the campus. They felt insecure, suspect, estranged, unrepresented, with no clear lines to those in power. Indeed, the gap between the agency and its constituency, and the Administration seemed to grow daily—with no end in sight. As the old saying goes, it ain't what you do, it's the way that you do it. Looking back, it's hard to see how the Administration could have done it less tactfully. Nixon surrogates with little empathy for the scientists they seemed to feel had grown fat and flabby at the federal trough, set about to manage NIH more closely. Impatient of scientific prerogatives, critical—except when NIHers won Nobel Prizes*—of spoiled intellectuals who seemed to be forever asking for more money, they held that the once proud, academically oriented NIH simply had to face tough 1970s budget realities and learn to do its research job as just another H agency.

Strong-armed, the officials of the Haldeman-Ehrlichman era moved in on the agency with all that green grass, all that brainpower, all that independence and all that money. When HEW Counsel Robert Mardian futilely rushed to court to enjoin a Viet Nam War protest meeting featuring Dr. Benjamin Spock on the NIH front lawn, he provided an example of their style (a jury later convicted Mr. Mardian as a Watergate co-conspirator). So did Alan May, the HEW secretariat's pink slip dispatcher, who walked into the Director's office, not only to tell him whom he must fire but report that he and a colleague had taken pictures of anti-Viet Nam War activists folding leaflets in an NIH building. More typical were the paper blizzards loosed in those early days on Building One, management-by-objectives directives under which NIH managers had to state their scientific goals, then frequently

---

*And even then praise was not easily come by. Although President Nixon was deluging the injured Washington Redskins quarterback with attention at the time the NIH's Christian Anfinsen won the Nobel Prize in 1972, the agency leaders had a hard time extracting Presidential congratulations. Finally, HEW Secretary Elliot Richardson hosted a small dinner at Blair House honoring Anfinsen and the two other Nobel Laureates at NIH; the White House was represented not by the President and Mrs. Nixon but by Mr. and Mrs. John Ehrlichman.

14

report progress in meeting them—a procedure which might have had some validity measuring numbers of services rendered in other Department social welfare agencies, but which at NIH benefited no one except recipients of Xerox corporation dividends, according to one who had to live with it. There was little understanding that medical research goals change as the search goes forward, one step builds on another—if you knew in advance where you would be on a certain date, you would not have to do the experiment that would get you there.

Or the obligatory chaperones from the HEW Secretary's legislative office downtown, who monitored NIH officials on visits to Capitol Hill like so many little boys and asked them to report routine telephone calls from Congressmen. ("I'm a registered Republican, but I've never seen anything like *that*" remembers former Deputy Director Sherman.) Or Secretary Weinberger's suggestion, which seemed to NIHers more that of a bookkeeper than an administrator who understood medical research, that NIH save money by asking Clinical Center patients to pay through third party insurance for services rendered. Or the attack on the peer review system, through which the Institutes had awarded grants successfully for decades. Some Nixon officials, especially at the Office of Management and Budget, saw peer review as a device through which the scientists were likely to make awards to friends through "old boy" methods. They regarded peer review meetings as expensive, and perhaps unnecessary. Why could not NIH administrators—who sat at desks which looked like Defense Department desks—make decisions the way Defense men do, without the advice of bunches of outsiders?

The NIHers returned the compliment. They bemoaned the "politicization" of a once above-politics agency. Speaking before a National Academy of Sciences symposium, former Director James A. Shannon observed for them that the Administration seemed to espouse the view that though NIH could continue to make day-to-day decisions, Presidential appointees would make the broader decisions at the political level. But these appointees, the NIHers felt, were ignorant of biomedical research method and substance and this ignorance resulted, among other unhappinesses, not only in interference with the peer review system, but in funneling funds into short-ranged "targeted" rather than more fruitful basic research; unbalanced pursuit of the quick cure for the popular highly touted disease, like cancer, without regard to current scientific opportunity; and emasculation of training support for the nation's future medical researchers. Despite an overall rise in the NIH budget, they said they did not have money enough to do all the things asked of them. As morale fell, it became harder to recruit staff for NIH positions at every level. "When I came here as a young man," a senior NIH physician recalled, "my friends thought I was coming to the Taj Mahal. Now they would ask, 'What the hell for? Not the money!' "

In the early days of 1974, three Democratic senators—Edward Kennedy of Massachusetts, Warren Magnuson of Washington, and Abraham Ribicoff of Connecticut—considered investigative hearings. In fact, Senator Ribicoff, a former HEW Secretary, convened an all day meeting to brainstorm NIH concerns (among those attending were former NIH directors Dr. James Shannon and Dr. Robert Marston, former top HEW officials like Secretary Wilbur J. Cohen and Assistant Secretary James Kelly and philanthropist Mary Lasker).

As the dark days of Watergate fell upon the Capital, as the disdainful Nixon managers fell from their pedestals, it was difficult to tell who was governing, and, in fact, if anyone was governing at all, much less what were the nuances of government health and bioscientific policies. A new NIH director, Dr. Robert S. Stone of the University of New Mexico, had to be given his fair chance. But Dr. Stone, a ponderously thoughtful, relatively obscure academician, had, perforce, to swim in dangerous waters, and far beyond his depth. At year's end, he joined the growing list of ex-NIH directors. Though he talked a managerial systems and subsystems patois (he had spent some months at the Massachusetts Institute of Technology's Sloan Management School), Dr. Stone's Department of Health, Education, and Welfare bosses felt he did not really know how to manage the Institutes.

Many medical scientists perceived the matter differently. The Federation of American Scientists called a press conference where the three NIH Nobel Prize winners as well as several other top NIH researchers vaguely deplored Dr. Stone's dismissal and the politicization of NIH research. Though they could name no specific issue on which Stone had taken a pro-NIH stand, they said he had been dismissed because he was an NIHer not an HEWer, and that NIH would be more independent if its director were a career, rather than a political appointee. Visiting scientist Dr. Jean-Marie Matthieu reflected the views of many less eminent NIHers: "Until a few years ago, NIH was largely independent of the executive branch of government," he wrote in the *Neue Zurcher Zeitung*. His interpretation was that President Nixon had appointed a manager responsive to him as Director "in order to bring the activities of NIH under his control." But Stone, "soon became infected with the spirit of freedom and independence prevailing at NIH" and lost his job.

1975 was a year of the search, and of the study. The Ford Administration completed a search for members of the President's Biomedical Research Panel which was mandated by the Congress when the Cancer Act was amended in 1974. Its report—a 15 month study of the NIH and ADAMHA (Alcohol, Drug Abuse, and Mental Health Administration), and their role in the whole federal health-research effort—was due in 1976. Some top health policy makers expected a great deal of this Panel. These included Senator Kennedy who deferred his promised exploration of NIH issues until the Panel had completed its study and made recommendations as to their solution. Another competing Congressional health

17

power, Chairman Paul G. Rogers of the House Interstate and Foreign Commerce Committee's Health and the Environment Subcommittee, has been less patient. Rogers launched a more modest investigation of his own, sending a young staff physician, Dr. David Banta, to spend four months at NIH, to interview, analyze, and form his own conclusions, with the help of several General Accounting Office staff members.

If this were just a fuss among several hundred bureaucrats in need of tender loving care, it would surely not be of national concern. But it is more than that. What is at stake here affects the heart, the multiple sclerosis, the arthritis patient—in fact, all who might profit from continuous, vigorous research and its application. Real questions as to the straightest road to medical progress are involved here, and real answers could have profound effect on the quality and duration of our lives.

To see what these questions are, and how they came to be asked, it is necessary to look backwards to the Golden Age of the National Institutes of Health, which coincided with the Golden Age of Medicine.

2. The Florence of the Renaissance

Dr. Shannon: "Mr. Rogers and members of the Committee, I hope my voice will carry, but I have long since lost a set of vocal cords."

Mr. Rogers: "I think we can hear you very well."

James A. Shannon, M.D. may have retired as director of the National Institutes of Health, and he may have lost his vocal cords. But the House Health Subcommittee Chairman Paul Rogers is right, everyone hears him very well. At 71 ("No, I'm not a living legend, you don't get to be a legend until you're 80.") he spends a great deal of time making himself heard: testifying before committees and commissions about the distinguished record of NIH, his fears for its future and for that of all medical research, writing a book, promoting his latest ideas. He does, as he puts it, get involved in a lot of things. He has come to personify the once happy marriage between the federal government and the bioscientific community.

Tall, erect, energetic, James Shannon gives the impression of someone full of the self-assurance, or hubris, that comes from years of running something significant and running it well. Weary of New York, where he served as special adviser to the President of Rockefeller University, he and his wife have returned to the Capital suburbs. Here, people recognize him— for instance, a young secretary as he arrives at a commission hearing, an elderly guard at the National Library of Medicine, where as a "scholar-in-residence" he works in a cubicle

19

reserved for him on the "B floor" stacks. ("Lord luv us, Dr. Shannon—you used to be head of NIH! You're looking great, sir.") Recently in the White House East Room, President Ford presented him and a dozen other top scientists with the National Medal of Science. Though this is the highest honor of its kind the United States Government can bestow, Dr. Shannon downplays its significance as an overture on the part of President Ford to the nation's disaffected scientists. He admits Vice President Rockefeller is favorably disposed to the world of science, and of universities, and he appreciates that Administration officials were sensitive enough to call him to ask if he would accept the medal if it were awarded. But he feels there has been no great change in Administration-NIH relationships since President Ford succeeded Richard Nixon; it's the Presidential Medal of Merit rosette he won in 1948 that he wears in his buttonhole.

Dr. Shannon cares about NIH and its constituency; some say he cares to the point of humorlessness. At the dinner-dance which crowned the Alumni Reunion weekend, he listened as the Ad Hoc Players, a quartet of health bureaucrats who have performed over the years at similar functions, ribbed NIH. For example:

First you get the forms from DRG*
Everything you need is furnished free
Dream up a project that's nice and fat
Then you add a bit of this and quite a lot of that . . .

Halfway through the show, Shannon interrupted the players, insisting that they stop. "I was furious," he remembers. "At a reunion of NIH scientists they were saying basically that the whole damn grant program was a rip off. I thought they should stop. I wouldn't sit down until they stopped." They stopped. Everyone still hears Jim Shannon very well.

NIH bureaucrats once tried to define a typical institute on one of those Parkinsonian administrative box charts, but

---

*Division of Research Grants

failed. No Institute is typical, each has its own personality, depending on the state of the art for which it bears responsibility, its array of substantive activities, its history, traditions, director and senior staff.

With an annual budget of some $325 million, and since 1972, its own enabling legislation carrying a three year authorization, the National Heart and Lung Institute (NHLI) is neither as old, as big, nor as rich as the quasi-independent $692 million Cancer Institute. Nevertheless, it is much bigger and more independent than Eye ($44 million) or Arthritis, Metabolism, and Digestive Diseases ($173 million), and very much a part of NIH, with separate intramural and extramural research programs. Its staff of 683, including 129 Ph.D.s, 151 M.D.s and three veterinarians (22 professionals have more than one doctoral degree) deals with the country's biggest killer—the heart and vascular diseases from which 28 million Americans suffer, and from which more than half of us die.

Like NIH itself, the Heart and Lung Institute has historically enjoyed outstanding leadership: Dr. James Shannon was scientific director before he moved to the NIH front office in Building One, as was Dr. Robert Berliner, now dean of Yale Medical School; both Dr. Donald Fredrickson, director of NIH, and Dr. Theodore Cooper, Assistant HEW Secretary for Health, were Heart directors* and a host of others trained and worked there before they went out to staff the nation's medical schools. Like NIH too, NHLI suffered a period of malaise in the early 1970s. For over two years after Director Cooper left for downtown and H, it was unable to attract the kind of director it wanted. (The last to turn down a search committee was Dr. Richard Ross, now Vice President of the Health Divisions and Dean of the Medical Faculty at The Johns Hopkins University, one of the three eminent heart specialists sent by Federal Judge John Sirica to examine Richard Nixon at San Clemente and determine if he was, as he

*Two former Surgeons-General were also Institute leaders, Drs. Luther L. Terry and William H. Stewart.

alleged, not well enough to appear in Court). With a salary ceiling of $37,800, a host of bureaucratic problems, and an insecure, hardly glamorous future, it was no longer able to compete for top staff in the inflated world of high medicine. Finally, in the fall of 1975, NIH Director Fredrickson handed the NHLI reins to a 38-year-old former associate, Dr. Robert I. Levy. Director Levy, a vigorous government career scientist-administrator, an authority on lipid metabolism who coaches Little League football weekends, now presides over an organization which reflects many of its sister Institutes' problems and concerns. NHLI can be a case in point.

The National Institutes of Health had its roots in a research laboratory founded at the Marine Hospital in Staten Island, New York, in 1887, and renamed the Hygienic Laboratory and moved to Washington in 1891. The name change was appropriate: in this era, most people died of infectious diseases like lobar pneumonia, or diphtheria or scarlet fever, and the only way to fight them was to establish "conditions or practices (as of cleanliness) conducive to health"—the Webster's definition of hygiene.

By the time the Congress transformed the Hygienic Laboratory into the National Institute of Health in 1930, set up the Cancer Institute in 1937, and certainly by 1944 when NIH got general legislative authority to conduct research, the whole pattern of disease had changed. A technology for controlling bacterial infection had come into being; generations of scientific investigators had identified tiny microorganisms called bacteria or viruses as a necessary cause of most infectious diseases. Effective prevention or treatment, culminating in the appearance of penicillin and the sulfonamides, followed.

Chronic diseases now emerged as the biggest killers and disablers. People freed by the new technologies to live longer lives suffered more illnesses, more complex, more difficult to understand — chronic diseases like cancer or heart failure induced by many factors, including our genetic makeup and

22

the way we live, not by one culpable germ. Still, the government's investment in biomedical research was a minor one. As 72 year old Senator Warren Magnuson of Washington, who introduced the bill that led to the creation of the Cancer Institute, reminded a Health Appropriations subcommittee recently: "Well, we started with $1 million, and if it had not been for that nice old lady donating all that land, why we never would have gotten off the ground." The Senator's mixed, but heartfelt metaphor, referred to Mrs. Luke Wilson and her prominent department store family (Woodward and Lothrop). They donated the major part of the present NIH Bethesda site to the government and thus enabled the agency to move in 1938 from modest quarters close by grounds where the John F. Kennedy Center for the Performing Arts now stands, and get a real start. The Wilson family added smaller parcels of land to the gift over the years, but still owns a house and more than three acres on the NIH campus.

Medical, like other energies, were concentrated elsewhere during World War II, and civilian medical research was put on a back burner. Afterwards, several Office of Scientific Research and Development military research contracts were transferred to the Public Health Service. With the support of PHS Surgeon General Thomas Parran, Dr. Rolla Dyer, the National Institute of Health Director, used them to start an extramural program, and these two unrolled grand plans for the greatest medical center in the world. Both the public and the Congress were amenable to the idea. Could not the scientists who discovered penicillin and the other miracle drugs which came into widespread use during the War find similar cures for the chronic illnesses? Now that communicable diseases were on the wane, could not the managerial genius that produced the atomic bomb find the cure for cancer or heart disease?

The lethal consequences of such illnesses were increasingly apparent to the Congress. Not only were constituents cut down in the prime of their careers, but so were prominent House and Senate colleagues, like Ohio's Senator Robert Taft,

23

a cancer victim not long after his unsuccessful effort to become the Republican Presidential nominee in 1952. A few years later, President Dwight D. Eisenhower, the victor in that election, suffered a massive heart attack during his first term, thus giving the public a more complete education in the symptoms and treatment of heart disease than it had had before. Will anyone who lived through that era forget the pro-exercise admonitions of elderly bicycle-rider Dr. Paul Dudley White, the President's physician?

The National Heart Act enacted in 1948, established the National Heart Institute and pluralized the name of the National Institutes of Health — and just in time. The National Institute of Dental Research was added that same year as were the National Microbiological Institute and the Experimental Biology and Medicine Institute.

The rush to form new institutes, one for nearly every class of important human afflictions, was on. The National Institute of Mental Health was established in 1949 and in 1950 the Omnibus Medical Research Act authorized the National Institute of Neurological Diseases and Blindness and the National Institute of Arthritis and Metabolic Diseases (which absorbed Experimental Biology and Medicine), and set the categorical nature of the Institutes in concrete. "Nobody ever heard of a person dying from microbiology" an influential Congressman was reported to have observed when the National Microbiological Institute became the National Institute of Allergy and Infectious Diseases five years later. Now Capitol Hill health aides make similar jokes about the National Institute of General Medical Sciences (NIGMS), the only completely non-targeted Institute, whose budget is always the most difficult to sell to Congress. President Harry S. Truman laid the cornerstone for the Clinical Center during the last days of his Presidency, and it opened in 1953.

The National Heart Institute (the Lung was not added until 1969) observes one alumnus, could be considered the

"Florence of the Renaissance", the medical research renaissance which flowered in Bethesda during the 1950s and 1960s. Fact and legend mingle here, but it is true that a combination of circumstances then made NIH the great and productive leader among the world's health research institutions. An expanding economy, a favorable political ambience, a consensus stemming largely from World War II technological success that scientific research can pay off big, and a set of remarkably effective health leaders in both public and private sectors, all worked smoothly in the Institutes' behalf.

The time was ripe; the postwar budget amenable; the cast of characters was small, select, and highly effective. The key committee chairmen in both House and Senate in the 1950s and 1960s seemed to the medical research administrator, heaven-sent. Senator Lister Hill of Alabama chaired both Senate committees crucial to medical research: the Labor and Public Welfare Committee, which handled health legislative authorizations, and the Appropriations subcommittee, which handled health funds—a concentration of power since unrepeated. The son of a surgeon, the relative of seven doctor cousins and brothers-in-law, he was named after the father of aseptic surgery, Joseph Lister, and had himself developed a deep abiding interest in health, and especially medical research matters. The late Congressman John E. Fogarty of Rhode Island chaired the House Health Appropriations Subcommittee for sixteen years during this same period. A former brick layer and union official, he was a self-made man who, while not as polished as the courtly Senator Hill, became his adept and knowledgeable equal in guiding his colleagues through the highly technical scientific wilderness toward generous support of medical research.

Two others, a man at NIH, and a woman outside of it, starred in this medical renaissance drama: Dr. James Shannon, who in 1955 became NIH Director, and whose intuitive political skill soon matched his medical research background;

25

and Mary Lasker, a very influential, passionately health-oriented philanthropist, who with her late husband, a millionaire advertising man, had founded the Albert and Mary Lasker Foundation and become interested in biomedical research as the straightest path to the reduction of disease and suffering, and in the federal purse as the only one fat enough to support it. Except for the Army Corps of Engineers, public administration specialist Rufus Miles points out*, there is probably no better example in the U.S. Government of the power of a "triangular political force" than that then exhibited by NIH (personified by Shannon), with the support of Congress (Hill and Fogarty) and outside pressure groups . . . (the "Lasker Forces").

Miles, an Assistant Secretary for Administration under six HEW Secretaries, Democratic and Republican, calls the relationship between the three a symbiotic one. A federal agency, he explains, develops simultaneous support from key members of Congress and outside pressure groups with an interest in the products and services of the agency. These key members find it to their own advantage to support the agency's programs and the pressure groups' interests, especially when they coincide with what they feel is the public interest. The pressure groups, in turn, are pleased when they get support from both key Congressmen and Senators and money-dispensing program agencies.

NIHers now look back wistfully and a bit romantically, at the golden age of this symbiotic relationship, when year after year Congress increased the President's request for their agency, often by many millions of dollars. These were the felicitous days, the happy days, when Dr. James Shannon could pick up the phone to recommend such and such a course of research action to the Congressional health appropriations czars. These were the days when potent NIH ally Mary Lasker, and her close allies, Mike Gorman, an irreverent Irishman, former newspaperman and promoter par excellence, and

*In *The Department of HEW*, Praeger Publishers, Inc., 1974.

Florence Mahoney, an astute lady with a talent for advocacy, argued the cause of health research in places of political power—on Capitol Hill, in the White House, and on the elegant Democratic dinner party circuit. So adept and thorough was Mrs. Mahoney at this particular *modus operandi* in the early sixties that she even played baseball with groups of HEW and White House insiders like Presidential Counsel Theodore Sorenson. A magazine article about her prowess headlined "Den Mother to the New Frontier" had to be killed when President Kennedy was assassinated.

It did not hurt that Mrs. Lasker knew how to contribute selectively to strong supporters in both Houses in their political campaigns. It did not hurt either that the alliance was a loose and informal one, as political scientist Stephen P. Strickland points out.* Its members never all sat down together and drew up or agreed on a set plan of action, and some even eventually developed definite reservations about each other. But they did toil vigorously and productively in the same vineyard, and if half of the Institutes had been put in place by the time Dr. Shannon became NIH Director, and if Mrs. Lasker, as she stresses to this day, was in Dr. Shannon's office only once or twice and talked to him seldom, she did speak often to her contacts on the Hill and her fellow operators spoke for her both to Shannon and to his Institute directors. Shannon and Fogarty were close. And, perhaps most importantly, in the NIH Director, the Congressional leaders had a scientist they could communicate with—and one who could talk to them for the scientific community.

No NIHer complained of politicization *then.* Each year the various National Institute directors would develop budgets telling the Administration and Congress what they could effectively use. After these estimates were reviewed by the NIH director and he modified or approved them, they were sent downtown to the Public Health Service Surgeon General's

---

*In *Politics, Science & Dread Disease,* Harvard University Press, 1972.

Office which normally, as Rufus Miles recalls, treated them like hot potatoes and passed them up to the Office of the Secretary as quickly as possible. Here, though NIH considered its relationship with some Secretaries—Marion Folsom, for example, or John Gardner—especially productive, they were usually cut and subsequently in the final Budget Bureau* competition they were cut again.

A predictable scenario followed. Congressman Fogarty had always done his homework; sometimes he even had a briefing breakfast with Director Shannon. At the hearing, Fogarty received the doubly-cut NIH budget with indignation (though the amount the Administration asked, as Rufus Miles points out, was always enough to carry forward the boost from the previous year, plus a little more). He would ask each Institute director how much money had been requested originally and could usefully be spent and then confront the Secretary, as the Administration spokesman, with the slashes which had been made in those funds. Then Mary Lasker and her colleagues would produce their citizen witnesses, distinguished and well rehearsed experts all, like Dr. Michael DeBakey of Baylor College of Medicine (Heart) or Dr. Sidney Farber of Harvard (Cancer), forcefully and thoroughly to inform the Committee of their cause. Fogarty was always able to persuade his colleagues to make significant increases over the President's budget. The same procedure was repeated in the Senate, where Senator Hill in his potent, gentlemanly way usually was successful in adding more.

The Heart Institute burgeoned as did all NIH. Heart's budget shot from about $16 million in 1950 (the President had requested $4.6 million) to $62 million in 1960 (the President had recommended $45 million) to $164 million in 1967 (the President had recommended $148 million). In those same years, the parent NIH budget went from $59 million to $1 billion.

---

*The Bureau of the Budget has now become the Office of Management and Budget (OMB).

Some say the Institutes got too much, too fast, from a cure-hungry, easy spending Democratic Congress. But looking back on their days as interns and residents, middle-aged cardiologists point to the dramatic improvements these medical renaissance years brought to their capability for treating and managing heart patients, and credit the Heart Institute and its ever expanding budget, with a large measure of that progress.

The Institute drew top scientists to Bethesda, both young and seasoned, excited by the prospect of doing excellent work with excellent people—pioneering, for example, in the catheterization of the left side of the heart (thus enabling surgeons to enter there, to diagnose, and perhaps to correct diseased valves or congenital defects) or in the treatment of hypertension with drugs, or in clarifying and diagnosing hyperlipoproteinemia—an excess of fatty substances like cholesterol in the blood which may lead to heart disease—thus starting the doctors down a new path urging people to control fats in their diets. It contributed leadership to the parent NIH as well as to the faculties of expanding medical academia beyond. Such are the achievements of its intramural research and training programs which Nobel Laureate Arthur Kornberg labeled of "stellar magnitude" at the Alumni Reunion. Another alumnus, Dean Stuart Bondurant of Albany Medical College, a member of the NHLI Advisory Council, goes so far as to label the NHLI program "one of the most distinguished and effective scientific enterprises in the history of mankind."

And across the country, where the Heart Institute supported 70 percent of all heart and blood vessel research "The NIH Connection" became the name of the game. No longer did investigators have to prove their worth to the Mellons or the Carnegies, but to NIH study groups, committees, and councils. In the Golden Years, the Heart Institute, like NIH itself, became the dominant source for research funding and an eminent success. Try to name the medical advance funded in those years without some Institute

29

support, from the heart-lung machine which maintains heart and lung functions during open-heart surgery, to the highly useful coronary profile (gained from the Framingham, Massachusetts heart studies) through which physicians can identify those susceptible to heart disease.

Now the surgeon enters where he never did before, correcting congenital heart defects. Man-made pacemakers and valves help the ailing pump to do its job; drugs control or prevent rheumatic heart disease, hypertension and heart failure; medical staff monitors patients with irregular heart rhythms, from the skipped beat to the serious standstill, in coronary care units. Some say the introduction of these units around 1960 in the United States cut heart attack deaths in hospitals by half.* Now heart attack patients spend two or three weeks in the hospital instead of four to six—an annual national savings in money—not to speak of pain, of some half billion dollars.

Still, 28 million Americans suffered some form of heart or blood vessel disease;** of the one million lost each year, between 200,000 and 250,000 are under 65. You can better manage the heart attack and its "sequelae", or results, than prevent it. For forty percent of heart attack victims, the first symptom is the last, they drop dead before they reach the hospital. Neither the Intramural Clinical Center nor the vast

---

*The difficulties in bioscientific evaluation are illustrated here. In Britain, a nation whose relative lack of affluence and National Health Service make for medical prudence in the widespread adoption of expensive new technologies, studies showed heart attack victims did just as well at home as in the hospital (initially in coronary care units). See *Acute Myocardial Infarction; Home & Hospital Treatment,* M. G. Mahler, et al, British Medical Journal, 7 August, 1971.

**Hypertension afflicted almost 23 million, coronary heart disease 3.9 million, rheumatic heart disease 1.7 million, stroke 1.6 million—some suffered more than one of these diseases.

array of Heart Institute-funded investigators had produced sure cures for this, or other chronic disease killers.

Heart disease research, like other disease research, had arrived at a fertile, but broad plateau. What's more, the Golden Years which had propelled it to this plateau, had not been golden for everyone. The turbulent sixties highlighted the inability of many families to gain access to acceptable health care, in remote rural areas as well as inner city slums. The very success of research had created a dissatisfaction — delivery of health services, availability of new discoveries, became the demand; perhaps some swollen NIH research funds could be more wisely spent in meeting it.

Pressures mounted in the mid-sixties, as leaders in the field and in the larger society outside challenged the Institutes to justify their size, their mission and the quality of their work. In the Congress, the Intergovernmental Operations Subcommittee chaired by North Carolina's Congressman Lawrence H. Fountain, in several reports, questioned loose administrative practices at NIH. But an unusually prestigious group appointed by President Kennedy's Science Advisor, Jerome Wiesner, and headed by Dr. Dean G. Wooldridge, in 1965 found NIH well managed, and after a comprehensive survey concluded that the scientific quality of the research it was buying with the federal tax dollar was good: "We suspect that there are few, if any, one billion dollar segments of the federal budget that are buying more valuable services for the American people than that administered by the National Institutes of Health."

In his National Library of Medicine cubicle a decade later, Dr. James Shannon recalled his and his former Institute Directors' two hour meeting with President Lyndon Johnson, a former heart attack patient himself, when John Gardner was HEW Secretary. The impatient President came through loud and clear: he wanted "results not research". Frustrated by the nation's uncomfortably low position on the international health totem pole despite huge investments in medical research

(18th in life expectancy for males, 11th for females; 16th in death of males in their middle years) and, at the height of the war on poverty, of the medical impoverishment of millions, the Democratic leaders of the sixties argued that emphasis should now be placed on testing and applying existing knowledge. ("A research discovery in the laboratory, until it is applied, saves mice, not men", HEW Secretary Abraham Ribicoff told a University of California Medical School graduating class in 1961.)

Mary Lasker and her allies had access to President Johnson and his staff; at the White House as on Capitol Hill, they had strongly advocated their belief in targeted research efforts and clinical applications — in trying to conquer dread disease by clinically testing what you were 60 percent sure of instead of waiting for that elusive 100 percent assurance. The President liked and appreciated Mrs. Lasker's vigorous style, he echoed her views when he spoke of zeroing in on targets by fully applying what was already known, of making sure no life saving discovery was locked up in the laboratory.

But you could talk, even argue with Lyndon Johnson. Dr. Shannon and his men asked for and were given time to analyze, to prepare, then to return with counter proposals. They felt they were able to convince him of their view: that theirs was a knowledge deficiency, not a management deficiency; that you cannot buy sure results; and that you cannot just wish solutions into complicated biomedical problems which must be solved step by step no matter how much money you spend, because they are quite different from military engineering problems like missiles development. Even with the Manhattan Project there could have been no success without the discovery of nuclear fission, and without the knowledge that pure physics and pure mathematics had accumulated during the two previous decades.

At the Heart Institute, for example, it was time to find out what basically goes wrong in heart disease. Then doctors could act as more than firemen, could prevent or even reverse the heart disease process, perhaps be able to put aside what Dr. Lewis Thomas, president of the Sloan-Kettering Cancer Center has since labeled the "halfway technologies"— from complex, costly specialized ambulances and electronic gadgetry, to the transplanted heart. It was time to find the root cause of chronic conditions like hardening of the arteries (arteriosclerosis), which over a life span of some 50 years clogs the blood vessels and brings on lethal heart attacks.

Johnson helicoptered out to NIH, and alluding to the Wooldridge report, called it a "billion dollar success". Then, almost before the researchers could breathe a sigh of relief, and while a new bright aggressive young Heart Institute director, Dr. Theodore Cooper, was taking hold, a Republican administration more difficult for NIHers to deal with came to power. This was an administration with some of the same agenda, but with a different philosophy, an administration emphasizing rigorous management and decreased government spending, skeptical of Democratic predecessors and suspicious of holdover scientist-managers as crypto-Democrats. It had little empathy with academic researchers, their casual dress, and their slow-moving scientific ways.

But it was an administration, nevertheless, like all administrations, which wanted badly to leave its own record of accomplishment. That, at the NIH, means the conquest of dread disease, and that costs money.

But where was that money to come from? Those marvelous large budget-producing paladins who might have continued to exercise Democratic power from Capitol Hill had begun to depart the scene. Congressman John E. Fogarty suffered a massive heart attack and died in his office in January, 1967. In 1968 Lister Hill, elderly, concerned for his sick wife, and in political trouble at home, retired from the Senate. Dr. James Shannon, now at mandatory retirement age, left the NIH Directorship.

For the first time, in 1968, Congress failed to up the Institutes budget, and in 1969 it dared lower it. As the economy

33

conscious Republicans turned to their tasks, the Golden Years at NIH — the years in which Americans and their representatives in the Congress seldom questioned the wonderful world of medicine and its practitioners and tried only to give them the means to do their job — were coming to a close.

3.

The Central Issue —1
Research and Results

In his Laboratory of Biochemical Genetics, Marshall Nirenberg bends over an inverted phase contrast microscope in his singleminded way. Tall, shy, and painfully soft spoken, he interrupts his work only to talk with a visitor about some of the events in and around NIH which have shaken the world of bioscience since 1968—the year, coincidentally, when he won the Nobel Prize for breaking the genetic code (the language through which genetic information, the stuff of life, is passed from one generation to the next). Now he studies how genetic instructions are assembled during the embryonic development of the nervous system, under the National Heart and Lung Institute umbrella. But his basic work was done at Arthritis and his laboratory is located in a building largely occupied by neurological workers. (The fundamental interdependence of the Institutes is illustrated also in the work of the two other Nobelists now at NIH: Christian Anfinsen of Arthritis used to head a Heart laboratory and Julius Axelrod of Mental Health, now organizationally outside NIH, grew up scientifically at Heart.)

The Nobel Laureate is likeable, and most modest. Though he heads a sizeable staff, he does his and his visitor's errands himself, goes to the coffee maker, finding it empty loses his own quarter in the coke machine. Though Dr. Nirenberg (Ph. D. not M. D.) has been offered more than twice his salary elsewhere, he stays at NIH largely because of the "wonderful" intellectual atmosphere: It's really like a university, with rich resources both in equipment and consulting expertise, seminars and evening courses, but without demands such as teaching chores or filling out grant applications. His wife, Perola, a neurochemist, works with his laboratory. Friends say the couple is intensely work-oriented; when he has a paper to write, he works straight through the night until the job is done, even if it takes 36 hours. They find him a "nice" man, a fine man, but when it comes to the science, a tough man.

His, Marshall Nirenberg explains, is basic research. People ask him if, because he works at the Heart and Lung Institute, he is working on heart and lung problems. But he cannot tell them precisely what clinical problems his findings might illuminate, or where they might lead. Perhaps they might lead to better understanding of cell communication in the circulatory system affecting hardening of the arteries, perhaps to a clue as to why normal cells begin to multiply malignantly: "It's difficult to categorize such work in terms of an organ or a disease. One really does not know. It's like a boiling soup; it changes rapidly, many options are available, we must have many independent investigators following many different leads."

"I used to think Mary Lasker was a little older than I am," mused one middle-aged high Heart bureaucrat, "now I think she's a little younger." With John Fogarty dead, Lister Hill and James Shannon retired, and a cadre of still untested Republican leaders in the White House, it was necessary for the indefatigable Mrs. Lasker and her allies in the cause of medical research to regroup, reassess, and find a different strategy.

It was equally necessary for the new Administration to find a different strategy. Not only did the continued escalation of NIH funding seem incompatible with Republican preachments of tighter management and more frugal government spending, it was also incompatible with rising demands from many quarters for post-Viet Nam budget reductions. If

NIH had enjoyed some success in the battles against disease, could it not enjoy more if it were managed more like the giant corporations which the new leaders regarded as paragons of efficiency?

The central question was, how to proceed? How to reach the rich, the solid, the long lasting research payoffs? How to find the straightest, and least expensive way to wipe out heart disease or cancer?

The bioscientists personified by Marshall Nirenberg felt then, as now, that stunning medical discoveries like the polio vaccine come not from huge, all out directed or targeted research efforts, but from the more diffuse "boiling soup" which he describes. They come from funding hundreds, even thousands of undirected individual investigators, each of whom initiates a search, then painstakingly, patiently follows his or her own tortuous research path. One, they reason, will reach the goal, perhaps alone, perhaps with others who have arrived on quite different paths, perhaps purposefully, perhaps quite by chance, while looking for another goal completely (they call this scientific serendipity).

This point of view, the point of view of the basic scientist, has been elucidated in a scholarly journal article* by two cardiopulmonary specialists, Dr. Julius H. Comroe, Jr. and the late Dr. Robert D. Dripps. *Question*: Have the dramatic discoveries of the past come from directed, targeted research, or from basic undirected research? *Answering examples*:

1) When Roentgen discovered x-rays, it was not to enable a cardiologist to visualize the coronary arteries of a patient suffering from angina pectoris; he was studying a basic problem in physics to determine the electrical nature of matter;

2) When Karl Landsteiner discovered blood groups, it was not part of a program to make blood transfusions safe; he was investigating basic problems in immunology;

---

*"Ben Franklin and Open Heart Surgery," *Circulation Research,* Volume 35, November 1974.

3) When Cournand and Richards passed a catheter into the heart of man, it was not to develop a new method of diagnosing heart disease; as primarily pulmonary physiologists they wanted to learn more about how blood and air are distributed to air sacs of lungs;

4) When Shackell developed the technique of freeze drying in 1909, it was not to preserve penicillin (there was no penicillin or plasma in 1909), but to find a better method of preventing water loss while he studied the water content of liver and muscle of steers;

5) When Clarke, a butterfly collector and amateur breeder, studied variations in the color of butterfly wings, he had no idea that it would lead to the discovery of the Rh factor in human blood;

6) When Davies and Brink devised an electrode to measure the partial pressure of oxygen, it was not to monitor blood oxygen in an intensive care unit; it was to measure oxygen consumption of resting and active sympathetic ganglia.

Another question: What had to be learned to permit the cardiac surgeon routinely and successfully to open the thorax, stop the heart, open the heart, restart the heart, and care for the patient to ensure full and speedy recovery (the clinical advance chosen in a poll by physicians and surgeons as the most important direct benefit to their patients since 1945)? *Answer*: Twenty five different bodies of knowledge, including anatomic and clinical diagnosis, transfusion, nutrition and intravenous feeding, asepsis, anesthesia and neuroblocking agents, anticoagulants, surgical instruments and materials, chemotherapy, pump oxygenator and wound healing. The heart surgeon hardly took a giant leap up the pinnacle of open heart surgery. Rather he climbed slowly, on steps laboriously chiseled by thousands of workers in many branches of science over the years.

But in the late 1960s and early 1970s the feeling grew that this climb had become too slow, too laborious and too laden with scientific perquisites. For one thing, the basic scientists were not adept at getting their point of view across. They knew it; pointing to the enormous public education job they had to do in convincing the public of the relevance of medical science to medical care, NIH Deputy Director for Science Robert Berliner in 1969 even suggested the equivalent of brief commercials on the label of each therapeutic measure, each dose of vaccine, each effective drug: "This is made possible by the research of Whozis and So and So; we trust you will find it effective and remember what research has done for you when you have occasion to influence the expenditure of your tax money."

Such commercials were not forthcoming. Instead, the policy makers in Washington heard arguments like those of the Lasker lobby, that the NIH investigators lacked a sense of urgency, their pace was too slow and cautious, their style too diffuse and undirected, irrelevant to present day clinical medical problems; their ambitions limited to the publication of papers to be read at scientific conventions in Atlantic City. After all, were the institutes National Institutes of *Health* or *Science*? It seemed NIHers would rather work on basic projects likely to bear fruit in 100 years than on clinical applications which might help at least some patients in pain today. If optimum good health for Americans were indeed the NIH mission, then the agency work should be more targeted, more responsive to the wishes of those Americans for the eradication of dread diseases. And in the opinion of at least some respected scientists the time was now ripe for an all out attack on cancer, the disease Americans fear most (though cardiovascular disease costs the nation twice as much as cancer and many more Americans die of it). Such an accelerated attack could not, the Lasker forces held, be launched by the National Cancer Institute, for its work was stifled by "six layers of HEW bureaucracy". Organizational changes were obviously in order.

The policy makers were persuadable. If it were not possible to get more money for all NIH, why not concentrate what they could get on one Institute? The idea of a targeted all-out war on cancer had wide appeal in the Democratic Senate, which the knowledgeable Lasker forces chose as the highly visible stage for the first act of the cancer drama, and where Senator Ralph W. Yarborough of Texas had replaced Lister Hill as Chairman of the Senate Committee on Labor and Public Welfare. In April of 1970, the Senate passed a joint resolution authorizing this Committee, with the help of an advisory committee, to report on the current status of the anti-cancer search and to recommend the measures necessary to ensure its success (an old Lasker forces device for providing two necessary ingredients: sound professional scientific advice and a prod for skeptical Republicans). A few months later, when the House and Senate passed a concurrent resolution expressing the unanimous sense of the Congress that the conquest of cancer is a "national crusade", the first guns in the War on Cancer were officially fired.

So on a Spring day in 1970, a letter came into the New York office of Benno C. Schmidt, managing partner of J.H. Whitney and Company (a capital venture firm), from his old Texas law professor, Senator Ralph Yarborough. To Schmidt, a portly, expensively tailored banker who retains more than a little of his folksy Texas charm, this letter asking him to accept membership on the new non-partisan Advisory Committee of Consultants on Cancer came out of the blue. Though he was a Republican from Texas, and a friend of Senator Jacob Javits, Yarborough's ranking counterpart on the Labor and Public Welfare Committee, and had served on the boards of the Sloan-Kettering Cancer Center and Memorial Hospital for Cancer and Allied Diseases in New York (as chairman), he was a stranger to the national politics of health research, and as he puts it now, did not even know President Nixon, not really.

But Benno Schmidt did know his way around the world of high finance now so closely tied to centers of political power; he owned a ranch together with banker David Rockefeller in Australia, and had worked, if not with Nelson, with Laurance on the Sloan-Kettering board, and he had more than a casual

40

acquaintance with a neighbor in Vail, Colorado, with whom he had skied and watched New Year's football, Gerald Ford. He was just what the cancer attack strategists needed for their Committee of Consultants (composed of 13 scientist-professionals and 13 laymen, including Elmer Bobst, President Nixon's "second father" and Laurance Rockefeller). When the Committee met in June, Senator Yarborough asked Schmidt to chair the group, and he displayed his considerable talents straightaway, calling on White House advisor George Shultz and advising the House leadership of the Committee's plans at a luncheon arranged by Vail neighbor (and House Minority Leader) Gerald Ford. He makes it sound so simple: "In order for something to happen, it had to happen in the House of Representatives too, and in the White House."

Schmidt reports the Committee of Consultants, especially its scientists, worked exceedingly hard. Yet before they could finish their job, Senator Yarborough was defeated for reelection in the Texas primary. Though his espousal of the popular cancer cause had not helped him politically, he strove as his Senate career drew to a close to promote the Consultants' report, delivered to him at the end of November. It recommended an all out, massive attack on cancer, and an independent National Cancer Authority directly answerable to the President to carry it out. Some said the recommendations did not have a chance, with Ralph Yarborough out of the picture.

But in January of 1971, a new health leader, Senator Edward Kennedy, now chairman of the Senate Health Subcommittee, picked up the reins. With Senator Javits, he introduced a bill embodying the Consultants' recommendations, a bill having 50 co-sponsors. Simply stated, the ensuing fierce legislative battle boiled down to this:

On the one side, the Senate version, establishing a separate independent cancer authority responsible directly to the President for a crash anti-cancer effort, backed largely by the "emotional" health lobbyists, some old-time Laskerites and

41

some new recruits (greatly helped by an urgent "write your Senator" appeal from syndicated columnist Ann Landers which produced hundreds of thousands of supporting letters).

On the other side, the House version, also enlarging and intensifying the anti-cancer effort, but retaining the Cancer Institute within the NIH structure, and backed by most NIHers, in and out of government and a newer lobby from the biomedical university community, represented by spokesmen from such groups as the Association of American Medical Colleges, the National Academy of Sciences, the American Hospital Association and faculty from the Harvard Medical School.

The Nixon Administration vacillated between the two, not wanting to be outshone in an attack on a deadly disease, especially by a Kennedy, but increasingly aware of the cries of alarm coming from the NIHers and their scientific supporters. At first the agency had lent the Consultants' Committee office space on the NIH campus, and staff time. But these outsiders did not consult with the NIH leaders in Building One, and as the debate built, as the Committee's plans to split their agency crystallized and the Senate began consideration of the Kennedy-Javits bill, NIH leaders grew more and more apprehensive. NIH Director Dr. Robert Marston, a virtual stranger to Capitol Hill, was seen there increasingly, lobbying against the Kennedy-Javits bill.

Naturally, the NIH administrators and working scientists resented the Senate's implication that they lacked a sense of mission and urgency, and that the new cancer effort could not possibly succeed unless it were taken away from them and given to a NASA-like (National Aeronautics and Space Administration) agency. More importantly, they grew ever more deeply convinced that the proponents of this proposal did not fully understand how profound its effect might be. Shannon argued that its enactment could be dangerously destructive and that scientific emphasis under the legislation "would be entirely determined by uncritical zealots, experts in

42

advertising and rapacious empire builders". He and other NIHers reasoned that the categorical disease approach had functioned smoothly because the Institutes were organized under a central NIH, administratively responsible not only for allocating resources among them and coordinating their activities, but for funneling research grant applications to them through the Division of Research Grants and the various study sections on cell biology or genetics or physiology. If the cancer program were cut away and other programs followed it, the balance between the Institutes, and between basic research and applied or directly disease-oriented activities, could be dangerously skewed. And it was from basic research that they felt all clinical applications must flow.

The Kennedy-Javits measure was compromised twice, first with a Nixon version submitted by a President who still employed a science advisor (the office was abolished soon thereafter) and to a much greater degree later, with the House version fathered by Health Subcommittee Chairman Paul Rogers, a legislator who was beginning to look as though he might try to fill John Fogarty's shoes. The NIHers had fared better in the House than in the Senate, despite renewed efforts on the part of the Mary Lasker-Benno Schmidt forces; the Rogers version of the measure sought to maintain an integrated research effort and keep the Cancer Institute within NIH.

Rogers had watched with interest as the NIHers' influence finally began to be felt. Three original scientist-members of the Senate cancer panel, Nobel Laureate Dr. Joshua Lederberg, radiologist Dr. Henry S. Kaplan, and oncologist Dr. Harold P. Rusch had broken from the group to encourage Senator Gaylord Nelson of Wisconsin in his efforts to keep the Cancer Institute within NIH. Nelson, whose interest in the issue was first aroused by medical scientists at the University of Wisconsin, cast a lone dissenting vote against the Senate bill when it passed in July of 1971, and it was a vote that was to echo down the years and be heard again.

43

In the end, the compromise measure which was enacted just before Christmas of 1971 ("a Christmas present for the American people" according to President Nixon), like most compromises, tranquilized many but completely satisfied few. It transformed the National Cancer Institute into an organization different from its sister institutes. It was still called the Cancer Institute, located on the NIH campus and in the Clinical Center, and participating in the larger agency's activities, including its basic research program.

But it had, as Director Frank Rauscher was to admit four years later, achieved a privileged status. It had its own access on high through a special mechanism worked out, largely by a conservative Republican member of Paul Rogers' Health Subcommittee, Ancher Nelsen of Minnesota: a special President's Cancer Panel monitoring its program and chaired by Benno Schmidt. It also had a presidentially appointed National Cancer Advisory Board, and an "end run budget" avoiding the HEW hierarchy and submitted directly to the President, or, in reality, his Office of Management and Budget. So it could win more money, positions and physical space than the others and command more attention for its disease and for itself; when other Institutes were told not to indulge in films and other such promotion "puffery", for example, the Cancer Institute was exempt. What's more, the NCI director, along with the director of the parent NIH, were no longer to be appointed by the HEW Secretary. They were to be appointed by the President.

The War on Cancer marked a turning point for NIH. The once proud and independent NIH had been treated like Peck's bad boy in the national arena. Though the outcome was not as unhappy as it might have been, NIH supporters charged the directorship had been politicized and they soon had evidence: though he had, eventually, sought to go along with the Administration's cancer bill, Director Dr. Robert Marston was dropped after the big Nixon win in 1972 when Mr. Nixon announced he was restaffing the government with executives of unquestioned personal loyalty.

Harsh language began to be heard in and around Building One. Out of office, Dr. Marston (now president of the University of Florida) implied the "jackass policies" of the Administration were destroying NIH. *Imbalance* became the code word for the War on Cancer program as the management-minded Dr. Robert Stone arrived as NIH director and the two deputy directors left their jobs—Dr. Robert Berliner in mid-1973, and a self-characterized "demoralized" Dr. John Sherman in early 1974.

Out in Building 36, where Marshall Nirenberg works, and in other laboratories at the Institutes and in the universities where NIH-funded investigators pursue the search, concern deepened and confusion spread. For the bioscientific community, the War on Cancer watershed epitomized a serious change, not so much in the amount of money available to all of NIH, which reached about $2 billion in 1972 (48 percent higher than in 1969) but in the way the extramural portion of that money is spent. Irvine H. Page, the Editor of *Modern Medicine*, sounded a shrill alarm in the pages of *Science** (often called the scientists' house organ). Warning that heart disease, our deadliest disease, was next in line, he wrote, "Scientists should be aware that this is a gut reorganization of basic biomedical science which deeply involves us all . . . Acceptance of whatever the legislative juggernaut demands seems inevitable. Much of the freedom of science is now being legislated away and we are approaching the Russian system of directed research."

In the fifties and sixties, the medical scientists explain, NIH monies were almost entirely allocated to individual researchers across the country through peer review, a two-tier system wherein grant applications are evaluated first by the applicants' expert peers according to scientific merit and then

---

*"Another Crusade", by Irvine H. Page. *Science,* 2 June, 1972.

by pertinent Institute Advisory Councils composed of non-government scientists and informed laymen, according to Institute and national priorities.*

Fifty-two committees or "study sections" primarily organized around the basic medical disciplines (like biochemistry, hematology, surgery, virology) review the grant ideas funneled to them through the central Division of Research Grants, recommend approval or disapproval and rate their recommendations on a weighted scale. The 10 to 15 members of a study section responsible for this primary technical review know their fields, know its needs, resources and scientific opportunities; they are the men and women best able to evoke the creative talents and energies of the nation's scientists: they could not be persuaded in any case to work full time for the government as project reviewers. The advisory councils decide how far an Institute's funds can go (in relation to its own and to national objectives reflected in its appropriated budget). Institute directors need Council approval to make research grant awards. Marshall Nirenberg sums up: "Peer review is just a tremendously good thing. Nothing is perfect, but this seems to be close to it. It really has worked superbly. As a matter of fact, it became a model for the world."

The War on Cancer watershed did not wipe out this technical peer review in 1971; far from it. The 1971 act, while exempting certain small grants from dual review, recognized the necessity of review for scientific merit; in 1974 the Cancer Act Amendments specifically reinforced the peer review concept. But criticism of the slow pace of the NIH *modus operandi* and its lack of frequent applicable results, reinforced the Nixon managers' skepticism of peer review (expressed first at the Office of Management and Budget, then in some quarters at HEW)—which, though it had never produced a

---

*The Councils turn down about 5 percent of the grants recommended to them by the peer review study sections.

major funding scandal, allegedly afforded too much travel to too many meetings and which had an ingrown incestuous pork barrel quality. Long after the Nixonians had left, a few Congressional critics continued to nag at peer review (although the chief critics—Wisconsin's Democratic Senator William Proxmire and Republican Representatives R.E. Bauman of Maryland and John Conlan of Arizona—concentrated their charges on a different sort of peer review at the National Science Foundation).

Importantly, the War on Cancer shifted the decision making process away from the scientists and away from the peer review of individually initiated research. More money began to be spent through two newer mechanisms: targeted contracts setting specific goals and not necessarily evaluated by groups of top research experts outside NIH through peer review, especially at the Cancer Institute; and various grants to groups of investigators at centers directed toward the conquest of specific diseases. These centers are chosen by review committees and usually involve site visits. The process may not be as intensive as is study section review of individual grant applications, since there are so many more scientific areas that have to be reviewed by a limited number of experts.

Adding insult to injury, the feeling grew that the professional-lay Advisory Councils to the Institutes responsible for the final review and recommendation (to the Institute Directors) of grant approval, had been downgraded. Rumors circulated that various Republican politicans had been asked to clear nominations to these Councils of "peer-statesmen", supposedly highly qualified educators and laymen. When former Vice President Spiro Agnew's friend Frank Sinatra was appointed to serve on the National Heart and Lung Advisory Council and then never showed up at a single meeting, the distinguished Dr. Julius Comroe, Jr., also then an NHLI Council member, complained vociferously on the editorial pages of *Science*.

There was no further Sinatra incident. Still, as the

47

Republican years proceeded, the Institutes, except for Cancer, found it harder and harder to get their own nominees for advisory councils approved downtown. Pressures for minority as well as for proper party representation on the Councils complicated and delayed matters. One Institute suggested an ear, eye and nose specialist be nominated for its Council; HEW countered by asking for a minority substitute. The Institute suggested a black physician from Tennessee, only to find his nomination unacceptable to top Tennessee Republicans. Naturally, the Institutes grew more and more up tight about suggesting names. Asked why he had no epidemiologist aboard his Council, one director said he could not find a Republican epidemiologist.

Only the privileged Cancer Institute, whose Board members were presidentially appointed, was consistently successful in getting a full complement of appointees. Only the Cancer Institute had Benno Schmidt aboard to insist on the prompt appointment of high caliber laymen and scientists, regardless of politics, race, sex, or geography. The NIH director's advisory committee had so many vacancies it could not produce the quorum required for a meeting. At the beginning of January, 1975, there were 75 vacancies among the 186 authorized council positions, by the following September, these vacancies had dropped to 56 and by December to 27 out of 190; by March of 1976, only seven vacancies remained.

Ironically, these vacancies were eventually filled not because the Administration had become less political but because it had become more actively so. HEW Secretary Caspar Weinberger had brought into HEW a 34 year old former Republican member of the Michigan legislature, William S. Ballenger. In January of 1975, Bill Ballenger took over as an assistant to the Secretary in charge of special projects—a euphemism for political clearance—and perhaps his most special project was the expeditious filling of the NIH council vacancies.

Ballenger is a personable but formidable young man

whose alarm-wrist watch sounds the end of interviews and proclaims him as a busy and well-organized executive. He remembers that he found a certain paranoia in his 20-person shop, once headed, in the early Nixon days, by Alan May. Ballenger reports he removed those who were possessed by suspicions that NIHers made up an "old boy" network, that they were resistant and could not be trusted to be accountable to the White House and the Administration. He adds that he replaced them with people whose style, like his own, resembles that of the President whose picture hangs outside his HEW door—Gerald Ford—open, candid, friendly and pragmatic in the belief that government can work and that the council vacancies could be negotiated with NIH.

Negotiations with NIH continued as Secretary David Mathews took over in late summer, but more slowly than Bill Ballenger had hoped. This was no state legislature: before he could even begin on the Director's Advisory Committee, he had to wait for the completion of a search for an eminent scientist to head NIH. He was also required to obey the mandates of the Federal Advisory Committee Act (P.L. 92-463) and an Executive Order (11769) which, however vaguely, commanded Government executives to consider the interests of minorities and women, as well as to balance points of view and function. He had to wait for NIH slates of candidates to filter up through HEW Assistant Secretary for Health Theodore Cooper's office and then through the career committee management bureaucrats "across the hall" before he could start negotiations with the Institutes.

Ballenger's account of these negotiations differs from that generally held at NIH. Downplaying the role of partisan party politics, he says his job is to try to persuade often inflexible people that "rather than have on a council a renowned scientist from New York City who is a 45 year old, white, Anglo-Saxon, Protestant male like maybe the other eleven members, why not have a black woman from Atlanta, Georgia, who may be equally or even more renowned but who doesn't happen to be a personal associate of some people at NIH?" On the other hand, NIHers, holding that prominent and well diversified lay people had always served on their Councils, looked at this espousal of the minority, feminist cause as sudden and disengenuous. They whispered that the Administration was using it as an excuse to gain control of the Councils—or at the least, to keep academicians suspected of liberal sympathies off of them.

October came; an article in *Science** magazine detailed the story of the NIH Advisory Council vacancies and Ballenger's role in filling them, and NIH dissatisfaction with the process. Senate health leaders reacted strongly. Senators Edward Kennedy and Jacob Javits, the ranking members of the Senate Health Subcommittee, fired off a letter to HEW Secretary Mathews. At year's end, during the debate on the National Heart and Lung Institute extension, Maryland's liberal Republican Senator Charles McC. Mathias, Jr. inserted the *Science* article in the record, and offered an amendment stipulating that all appointments to advisory committees under public health legislation "shall be made without regard to political affiliation."

In his HEW office, Bill Ballenger reacted skeptically. To him, the Senators' complaints seemed meaningless and ironic. After all, the Congress is the ultimate in political bodies; its members routinely suggest candidates for councils, committees and other offices. Though he did not like to say "hypocrisy," the word did spring to his mind when he considered that Senator Javits without question was the biggest voluntary supplier of candidates: "It bears little relation to reality. It's just a game that's being played."

Whatever the game that was being played, and whoever was playing it, the basic scientists like Marshall Nirenberg were right. The tide had turned away from them as apolitical decision makers. The tide had turned away from individually-initiated research chosen through a dual peer review system.

In fact, it seemed to be moving in the opposite direction.

---

*"NIH Advisory Committees: The Politics of Filling Vacancies", by Barbara J. Culliton, *Science*, 31 October, 1975.

4.

The Central Issue—2
Relevance and Accountability

Underneath the operating room dome, they wait: patient, assistant surgeon, nurses, technologists, anesthesiologists, observer physicians—green gowned, masked, capped. Everything is ready, the patient completely covered with a drab green sheet, anesthesized and "cannulated" or hooked up to the heart-lung machine, her dark red blood flowing through its plastic tubes, her chest opened. Only her heart can be seen through a square hole in the sheet. It pumps very slowly: The Tell Tale Heart. Dr. Michael Ellis DeBakey enters scrubbed and capped, slips into the gown a nurse holds for him, moves to the patient's right side to begin the critical procedure: stitching a large vein from the leg into the aorta which carries the blood away from the heart, and then into one of the small blood vessels feeding it, thus bypassing or detouring the damaged section and permitting the body's vital pump to do its work. It is 8:30 a.m.; DeBakey has been at work at Methodist Hospital in Houston since 6:30.

Watch now, you stand at the pinnacle of American medicine. Exquisitely dextrous, absolutely competent, head of a perfectly orchestrated team accustomed to defying nature and challenging mortality, the surgeon places the vein around his patient's heart, suturing carefully, concentrating completely on the task. A computer monitors the patient's functions, flashing the essential information onto a television screen above—blood pressure, venous pressure, blood chemistry, temperature, ECG; pump technologists monitor the heart-lung machine. A fully trained cardiovascular surgeon works on the other side of the patient; he will close her chest wall and supervise as she is taken to the intensive care unit. Four such teams work in tandem, permitting DeBakey to do between eight and twelve and perhaps as many as fifteen operations a day, sometimes as now, just stepping in to do the critical procedure, in more complex cases, staying from start to finish.

It is 9 a.m.; DeBakey races the clock. Downstairs, his patient's family awaits him; he tells them the operation went well, then turns them over to his "Cardiovascular Coordinator", Nurse Sylvia Farrell (a most able lady who is not above hanging pictures of grateful movie star patients on her wall or reminiscing fondly about the time when Lyndon Johnson walked into her office unannounced, or when she gave Astronaut John Glenn a flu shot). Sixty-seven now, the country's best known surgeon gets up each morning between 4 and 5 a.m., works at his desk for an hour or so, then drives to the hospital in either his Ferrari or his Maserati sports car. The sign beneath the nameplate on his office reads "Director, Cardiovascular Research".

In this office, between operations, or in his Presidential quarters at Baylor College of Medicine close by which he uses far less often, DeBakey writes letters, dictates, or attends meetings. A Washington bureaucrat recalls one afternoon's meeting with him interrupted five times so that he could climb the stairs to the operating room (faster than the elevator). On an especially heavy day, he may not finish until 10 p.m. What's more, he often travels out of town; he leaves Houston this afternoon to give a series of lectures and demonstrations in Iran, on the way he will stop off at Williamsburg, Virginia for an editors' conference. Twice, in the past several weeks he has flown to Washington, once to testify before a Presidential panel, once to attend an NHLI Advisory Council meeting.

He maintains a teaching schedule, and as an extra

52

dividend brings a group of "tremendous" high school science honors students to work with his staff in the laboratories every summer. ("I have patients who are willing to give me money for things like that".) He is intensely involved in his work, enjoys it more than any hobby. Recently, he married a young German actress and reports his new wife is a "wonderful girl" who believes in what he is doing. Some publicity-shy physicians look askance at Michael DeBakey, as they might look at any globe-trotting, politically active surgeon who has been featured on Time Magazine's *cover. But most now admit that more than any other clinical investigator, he has somehow found the extra time and energy to step out of the operating room and the laboratory to tell the story of medical research, with all its problems and possibilities, to the public, and to do so with skill and enthusiasm. He dates his insight as to how the federal government, and especially the NIH might enhance the health of the American people to his service in Washington during and after World War II, first in the Army Surgeon General's Office and then working for the National Research Council developing a clinical research plan for the Veterans' Administration, and for the Hoover Commission's medical task force. Now he heads the first National Heart and Blood Vessel Research and Demonstration Center (or "Supercenter") at Houston—a five year, $13.3 million program funded by the National Heart and Lung Institute.*

"We are Cancer watchers", says the prescient Jerome Green, the NHLI's extramural chief, "We are Number Two, we learn from Cancer's mistakes". No one at the Heart Institute or in its constituency outside learned more from the cancer theatrics of the early 1970s than the Institute's own director, Dr. Theodore Cooper. Even before the cancer Committee of Consultants made its report calling for an all out War on Cancer, he convened a blue-ribbon task force of scientists and physicians (no Elmer Bobsts or Frank Sinatras here) to develop a long ranged plan to combat arteriosclerosis or

53

clogging of the arteries.* If heart disease, the nation's biggest killer, was to be next on the politicians' list, the Institute would retain the initiative, not yield it to Congressional advisory committees whose credentials might be more political than medical. If heart disease research were to be more relevant, more accountable in terms of producing cures for the taxpayers who were footing the bill, its tasks would be influenced primarily by scientists and physicians.

Predictably, the Arteriosclerosis Task Force recommendations delivered to Dr. Cooper in June of 1971 were different from those of the Committee of Consultants on Cancer. They did not mention removing the Heart and Lung Institute from under the National Institutes of Health umbrella or weakening the NIH structure in any way. Instead they suggested that NHLI develop, promote and support "a national coordinated comprehensive program" for the prevention and control of arteriosclerosis, stressing the acceleration of both basic and applied research, the efficient application of its results, and an effective health education system. Pointing out that the anti-arteriosclerosis effort had probably been slowed unnecessarily because it was fragmented into small programs at many universities and hospitals, the task force specifically suggested the establishment of National Centers for Prevention of Arteriosclerosis at several medical centers—centers in which cardiologists, surgeons, pathologists, biochemists and other professionals could jointly mount an interdisciplinary attack on the disease. Their other recommendations included smaller

---

*Arteriosclerosis, commonly called hardening of the arteries is a generic term which includes a variety of conditions which cause the artery wall to become thick and hard and lose elasticity. Atherosclerosis is a kind of arteriosclerosis in which the inner layer of the artery wall is made thick and irregular by deposits of a fatty substance which project above the artery's inner layer and decrease its diameter. (from A Handbook of Heart Terms, NIH, U.S. Department of Health, Education and Welfare, 1975.)

Cardiovascular Disease Clinics within the framework of existing medical care, to screen those people most at risk or those most likely to fall victim to the disease.

It is important to note that the center concept embodied in this set of recommendations dates back to World War II days, when, according to Dr. Michael DeBakey, concentrated centers of medical expertise (neurosurgery, or orthopedic surgery—or even centers within centers like intensive care) had to be established because of shortages of specialized personnel. Testifying before a House Appropriations Subcommittee a dozen years before the Arteriosclerosis report, DeBakey suggested that this center concept be applied to help the nation realize its medical research goals. He told the legislators he would like to submit for their consideration what he considered to be "the most impressive concept for actuating a concentrated attack on cardiovascular disease . . . the establishment of research centers that provide a broad and stable organizational framework in a proper intellectual and scientific environment and (which) can bring together the best of our scientific researchers in a stimulating intellectual group wherein their ideas may have an opportunity to cross-fertilize and germinate . . . "

President Lyndon Johnson made DeBakey head of a Commission on Heart Disease, Cancer and Stroke (Mike Gorman served as staff director) and the mid-sixties saw the beginnings of a system of federally-sponsored special heart, cancer and stroke programs. Originally they were visualized as a network of regional centers of excellence for research, training, and patient care, centers which would demonstrate new technical advances in their own areas. But they became entangled with the fears of organized medicine, then busily engaged in fighting Medicare, about further enlarging the federal role in the delivery of health care beyond that of pure research. As a result, the law establishing the Regional Medical Programs defined them loosely, and they became, with few exceptions, nondescript large grant programs (administered at first by NIH, and later by the H services administration), focused on the continuing education of physicians. With the enactment of a new health planning law in 1974, these programs began to be phased out.

But the centers of excellence concept survived. DeBakey considers it certainly not the only approach to research problems, but one of a number of fruitful approaches in a pluralistic system. At Baylor, he obtained one of the Heart Institute's first large program project grants (PPGs) for multi-disciplinary cardiovascular research. Looking back, he remembers that such group grants did not enjoy much popularity fifteen years ago; individual research scientists feared they would be dominated or directed in research groups. On the contrary, DeBakey insists, they found at Baylor that they were strengthened by "collateral support."

The legislative pulling and hauling which preceded the enactment of the National Heart, Blood Vessel, Lung and Blood Act of 1972 was a mini-battle, compared to what preceded the enactment of the War on Cancer Act. For sure, diverse bills were introduced, including several which would have removed Heart-Lung from NIH and placed it directly under Presidential control. House Committee on Interstate and Foreign Commerce Chairman Harley Staggers (to whom Mary Lasker and her colleagues had turned when Health Subcommittee Chairman Paul Rogers began to move away from the all-out Senate Cancer bill) in January 1972 offered a similar measure for Heart, including the Institute Director's appointment by the President and end-run budget access. Another similar bill was introduced by Congressman Claude Pepper, a longtime Lasker friend, who, as a Senator in the forties had been a leader in the establishment of NIH and an original cosponsor of the National Heart Act. In addition, his bill called, like the Cancer Act, for the establishment of a three member Presidential Heart and Lung Panel to oversee the program and a Presidentially-appointed National Heart and Lung Board.

But time had passed, experience had been gained, the NIHers had had their say; this was a different ball game. Fewer Madison Avenue techniques invaded the bioscientific bailiwick; there was a blessed (to the NIHers) absence of pro-Big Heart Bill advertising in Congressmen's hometown newspapers. The final definitive measure, this one the product of a happier Kennedy-Rogers union than the first, reflected (and indeed specifically acknowledged in the Senate report) the legislators' access to the set of recommendations made by the Institute professionals themselves, articulated especially by the Arterioscleriosis Task Force. These included the balanced expansion of both basic and applied research, the establishment of National Research and Demonstration Centers and the retention of the Institute and its advisory board within NIH.

It reflected too, the astute Dr. Ted Cooper's strong ties with both the heart-lung professional community and with his mentors in Building One, and the fact that its lobbying support was a world apart from that of the emotional cancer lobbyists. The newer lobbyists for medical academia, like the Association of American Medical Colleges, were arguing more vociferously than they had before for maintaining the scientific togetherness and integrity of NIH, and there were more of them.

What's more, though the American Heart Association, the largest and most prestigious group in the field, definitely wanted a bigger and more expensive heart research effort, and made its wishes known on Capitol Hill, it could not have been tempted toward an extreme War on Cancer position. In the eyes of a Lasker lobbyist like Mike Gorman, the American Cancer Society did not emerge from that war as the most aggressive possible proponent of the cause, for in the end, it did not even support the all-out Senate measure. But to most it seemed and seems a gladiator compared to the more cautious American Heart Association (in whose counsels laymen have a weaker voice). Though the AHA raises some $60 million each year—$16 million for research, usually coordinated with that of NHLI; the rest for such activities as public education and scientific meetings—it is politically low-key, and not especially government or Washington oriented. In fact, it moved its central offices from New York City to Dallas, Texas in the summer of 1975 and keeps tabs on Washington matters through a part-time Washington lobbyist and a staffer who visits the Capital periodically.

Support for the moderate Kennedy-Rogers approach came too from the medical scientists and physicians represented by such professional organizations as the American College of Chest Physicians. True, they were able to obtain the specific priorities for lung and blood research originally proposed in a bill introduced by Minnesota's Senator Walter Mondale—15 percent of the NHLI budget for each—and NIHers would rather have set these percentages themselves, according to scientific opportunity. But this was the only political meddling in NHLI affairs which appeared in the Act, and it came from medical scientists themselves, not from outsiders. However politically appealing the priority it smells most sweet to NIH when it is set by peer-colleagues.

So the Heart and Lung Institute stayed within NIH, and NIHers reasoned the decision-making pendulum perhaps was swinging back a bit in their direction. It became a bureau with much more money and an authorization which, like the Cancer Institute's, must be reviewed every three years. Its mandate was greatly broadened, to include not only new fields, but new expanded activities stretching across the whole research spectrum. Basic science was not to be ignored; on the contrary, its practitioners were to be increased and their work intensified. They were, however, to be joined by a host of others unknown to their grandfather-medical scientists, from administrators of clinical trials and computer programmers to media specialists.

The Congress directed the Institute in the National Heart, Blood Vessel, Lung and Blood Act of 1972 to prepare a five year plan to carry out a broad program of research. And it authorized up to thirty "supercenters"—15 for heart, blood vessel and blood diseases, 15 for chronic lung diseases—each of which would cover the whole research spectrum. Later, this was to be defined in the NHLI five year plan in this way:

1. The acquisition of new knowledge;
2. The testing and evaluation of existing knowledge;
3. The application of existing knowledge.

One was already underway; it was necessary to step up number two and to launch three from the beginning.

Budget realities cut these grandiose plans by ten. Today there are not thirty supercenters, but three, in each of the NHLI's areas of concern: heart and blood vessel, lung, and blood. Forty seven academic health centers and non-profit organizations competed for these awards. Dr. Michael DeBakey's Baylor College of Medicine was selected as the first National Heart and Blood Vessel Research and Demonstration Center after NHLI peer review committees averaging 18 specialists each, had visited 25 applicants, staying an average of 4 days. (The smaller lung disease research and development center went to the University of Vermont, the still smaller blood center to the Puget Sound Blood Center in Seattle, Washington.)

Ordinarily, when such a government grant is announced the local newspapers carry a dry five-line story recording the event. In contrast, both Houston newspapers front-paged the news of the development of the city's new center, and on July 27, 1974, the *Houston Post* editorialized "Houston is honored." Pointing out that the new Research and Demonstration Center seemed likely to involve all of Houston in a "vast complex plan of research, demonstration, education and prevention," the newspaper observed that "the stern and dedicated scientist alone in his laboratory is a figure out of the past century."

This may be poetic license. Just as the National Heart and Lung Institute, like all NIH, still devotes the greater part of its research budget to the individual investigator in his laboratory—some as stern and dedicated as Dr. Marshall Nirenberg, some not—so does the Baylor Supercenter. But it is true, that in this new center, set up under the 1972 Heart, Blood Vessel, Lung and Blood Act, the scientist is not and cannot be a loner. His work is necessarily part of a broad attack on cardiovascular disease; thus he has been joined by specialists who might make the old fashioned scientific purist shudder, like communications people or nutritionists or ambulance firemen.

What is more, the effort is taking place not only on the huge Texas Medical Center campus, which numbers Baylor College of Medicine and Methodist Hospital among its 29 institutions, but out in the Houston community, in its public schools and in a network of seven clinics which care for low-income Black and Mexican Americans. As the Supercenter's public education director Frank Weaver puts it: "Most medical research scientists have traditionally operated in a kind of hotel fashion—their own space, their own territory, their own budgets—they do their thing and so be it. They communicate through their respectable professional journals and meetings; they have not had to expend as much energy relating their work to the work of others, and capitalizing on the human resources of academic medical centers. We're trying to change that and we're trying to evaluate the change and that's a difficult thing."

The returns are far from in on this five year $13.3 million Research and Demonstration Center. But a brief look at it well into its first year may elucidate some of the problems and possibilities of such an effort as well as the words and phrases bandied about in Washington when health administrators and legislators confront research and health care problems: "basic" or "applied" or "continuum" or "translation gap".

Like its leader, the Baylor Supercenter is vigorously targeted, which means it is using taxpayers' money not to study just what happens to intrigue individual investigators, but to achieve definite goals. "No doubt about it," states Dr. Michael

60

DeBakey, "arteriosclerosis is now the main challenge for heart disease research." Is there a solution on the horizon for this disease? "Sure. Look, it is important to accept the notion that every disease has a specific cause and when you find that cause you can prevent it. History has demonstrated this effectively."

Another DeBakeyism which underlies the Supercenter, a simple concept, the surgeon admits, perhaps deceptively simple: "If Johnny gets lost in the woods and you send ten men to find him, they'll find him in a certain time. But if you put 100 men in that same area, they are going to find him ten times sooner." At Baylor almost 70 percent of the $2.6 million first year budget has been put in the Division of Basic Research— finding Johnny through the acquisition of fundamental new knowledge about the causes, prevention and treatment of cardiovascular diseases and their complications. An old bio-scientific saw is reflected in this nomenclature. Here, as among scientists elsewhere, basic research is like motherhood; no matter how closely involved they are with research targets, investigators prefer to be for it and to be labeled "basic". (An NHLI official recalls one university investigator who objected, during an administrative reorganization, to having his basic lipid chemistry grant transferred to a specifically named, and therefore "applied" arteriosclerosis unit.) Both basic and clinical research are represented in the Supercenter basic division; both represent a continuation of basic and clinical research supported over the past fifteen years under Heart and Lung Institute interdisciplinary grants, first a cardiovascular program project grant (PPG) to Dr. DeBakey and more recently a specialized center of research (SCOR) grant to Dr. Antonio M. Gotto, Jr. Dr. Gotto, another of the research investigator-stars trained like NHLI Director Robert Levy in the Intramural program under Donald Fredrickson, is the Supercenter's scientific director to whom DeBakey has delegated its day-to-day management.

The white-coated scientists working in the research division do not look too different from those in other busy cluttered university labortories. Nor is their work too different. As research scientists, for example, Dr. Gotto and his colleagues in the lipids section, are investigating how proteins carry lipids, or fatty substances. Somehow, the protein-boats in the blood bind these lipids, and they are deposited on the blood vessel walls, where, in some people, they can gradually collect and clog the passageways. Once the scientists know exactly how these lipids are transported, Dr. Gotto reasons, they will be on their way to finding a way not only to prevent their deposit on the vessel walls, but to reverse the clogging process. Then doctors could hopefully discover a way to pull the lipids out of the walls, washing out clogged arteries, and cholesterol-conscious dieters could eat all the eggs and drink all the milk they want. "We are trying to do good basic science," Gotto explains rather defensively. "We are investigating the basic mechanism of lipid transportation in the blood; we publish our papers in professional biochemistry journals, not special heart journals. But we are working within a center which is heart disease-oriented and we hope our work has a potential clinical application. Just because it is targeted does not mean it is not quality research."

The search in all seven of the Division of Basic Research sections—Morphology, Myocardial Biology, Cardiology, Surgery, Immunology and Blood Resources as well as Lipids—involves both basic and applied or clinical work to different degrees. Lipids, for example, is mostly basic but it is in some measure clinical because most of the studies there deal with human material. As principal investigator of the largely clinical Surgery section, Dr. DeBakey monitors the effectiveness of cardiovascular surgery and is working to develop and refine new surgical procedures and surgical support systems as well as to reduce post-operative complications. His group is also studying where the sac-like clots in coronary by-pass patients originate—in which vascular beds they first balloon—and the possible reasons why some develop slowly, over the years, and some bulge the vessel walls quickly, overnight.

Though they reflect nearly 70 percent of its budget this year, these research programs alone would not make the center "super". What has made it so is the addition of the two new research areas mandated by the Heart and Lung Act of 1972—Demonstration and Control (22 percent of the first year budget) and Education (8 percent). These reflect an increasing impatience in the Congress with the pace at which the fruits of research reach patients—an impatience parochially known as the translation gap. (A Senate Appropriations Committee report directing all NIH to try to close this gap and speed knowledge from the laboratory bench to the patient's bedside has been referred to around the agency front office as "the gospel according to Senator Magnuson".)

In the early 1970s, for example, physicians knew how to treat and control most hypertension—or high blood pressure—which may lead to increased heart size and kidney damage. But half of the estimated 23 million Americans suffering from this disease did not know they had it; only half of those who did know it were in treatment, and only half of these, or some 3 million patients were taking the right medicines, eating properly, and doing what the doctor said to keep the disease controlled. In the same way, doctors know that some people run a greater risk of falling victim to heart disease if they eat diets rich in animal fats or smoke excessively. But they feel they have not been especially successful at helping them change such lifestyle habits; on the contrary, there has been a rise especially in the number of women and teenagers who smoke in the United States.

Historically, the most successful disease prevention and control programs like mosquito spraying or rat control or mass immunizations have been directed at communicable diseases and most often done for people, or in the case of immunizations, to them. Now disease prevention, particularly chronic disease prevention, requires that patients enter into a therapeutic alliance with their doctors. They need, not just to become aware of the necessity for certain actions, but to take such actions for themselves. The Houston Supercenter has

63

begun a series of intriguing community-oriented research projects to find out how this might best be accomplished.

Take the smoking project. The best way to tackle the smoking problem, says behavioral scientist Dr. Richard I. Evans of the University of Houston, is to work not with adults addicted to the habit, but with young people who have not yet become addicted. Under psychologist Evans' direction, the Supercenter smoking research study has been carefully designed to teach 5th through 12th graders to recognize societal pressures to smoke and learn how to spurn them. "If we could keep just five percent of our students across the country from starting to smoke," Psychologist Evans explains, "we could save more lives than we could through all the palliative medical actions we take for them throughout their lifetimes. And that's a conservative estimate."

Seventh graders in the Houston public school system, or about 750 twelve year olds have been involved in the pilot for the larger study. Investigator teams visit them in their classrooms, showing them audio-visual films and leading them in "focused" discussions centered around three themes: the pressures their peers put on them to play it cool and smoke; the more subtle pressures their smoking parents may put on them; and the media ripoff or pressures society puts on them through cigarette advertisements, appealing to normal human desires to stay young or beautiful. The teams return to the classrooms later to find out from the students how they think they are doing. They do not seek to scare the twelve year olds with gory heart failure or lung cancer pictures, but to ask them to make their own public statements as to how to achieve independence—how to be their own men and women, and not just sheep in a herd—by positively refusing to smoke.

Two measures are being used to test progress. One is a 36-item questionnaire. The other is the first practical offspring of the Supercenter marriage between behavioral and basic or medical "hard" scientists. Because Evans, whose experience includes investigation into preventive strategies in oral hygiene, feels you cannot depend on fallible human beings to report accurately on their own behavior, he asked Baylor Chemistry Professor Evan Horning if he could develop a physiological measurement for smoking like the red dye used in dental studies to determine how well people brush and floss their teeth.

Horning said he thought he could, and using mass spectroscopy, a process which separates substances by mass, he did devise a test detecting the levels of nicotine in saliva (preferred to a urine-detection test which had turned off some students in drug studies). The test is given before the students enter the smoking project and periodically thereafter, to support or disprove their own questionnaire answers. Five different combinations of independent variables or experimental conditions are compared, and two control classes receive only the pre-test and one post-test. It might be that just knowing you are going to be tested—like just knowing you are going to be weighed in an obesity program—might change your smoking habits.

In a similar program, Supercenter investigators are trying to find out the most effective way to help people modify the fatty diets which, like cigarette smoking, are strongly associated with increased susceptibility to coronary heart disease and its complications. Here too, they use a physiological measurement—testing peoples' blood lipid levels—to see how they respond to various sets of conditions.

Many in the health research establishment say they are not comfortable describing such research as control and demonstration projects. Assuredly, the Supercenter smoking and diet modification programs seek to find ways to control bad health habits. But what about that ambiguous term "demonstration"? You cannot demonstrate something you do not already know, and if you already know it, why does it have to be researched and evaluated?

The Supercenter Control and Demonstration Division,

headed by Dr. Carlos Vallbona, head of Community Medicine at Baylor, is building on a relationship already established with the Harris County Hospital District's network of seven neighborhood clinics to demonstrate advances worked out in its own, or other laboratories. Baylor has developed a data base for these clinics: health/illness profiles of some 7,400 of the 70,000 registered clients, which can be used in Center studies. Every time an investigator wants to know exactly who, for example, has hypertension, or who has suffered both arteriosclerosis and stroke, he has only to ask the computer for names and addresses. First priority will be given to a hypertension study comparing various medical protocols (or standard sets of procedures) to find out which works most effectively in managing hypertension patients. Obesity may be next on the list.

A slightly different demonstration also hooks onto an ongoing community program: the Houston Fire Department's ambulance service which carries heart attack victims to the hospital. These ambulances, equipped with special telemetering equipment enable doctors in the hospital to monitor patients while they are still en route, and to instruct trained firemen in their care. Supercenter investigators will try to find out how effective this system is in reducing the large percentage of cardiovascular deaths that occur before heart attack victims ever reach the emergency room, and at what cost. If the ambulance system does not work well enough, says Scientific Director Gotto, it may be because these people and their families do not call the ambulance quickly enough: It's the first 15 to 20 minutes which make the difference; not realizing this, most procrastinate, trying this and that, waiting for the pain to go away.

Which brings the Supercenter research story back to education—a thread which runs throughout its structure. The Public Education section started its job by conducting a mass survey of Harris County to find out how its immediate public felt about heart disease and the chief risk factors involved, like smoking; what its health needs and priorities were; what media sources it turned to for health information. A second study attempted to define the role mass media "gatekeepers" can play in health education (these turned out to be food editors more than medical or science writers). Working with these survey results, and with other section investigators, the communicators will develop education programs for Houston, such as the one planned to emphasize the recognition of heart attack symptoms and the importance of calling an ambulance quickly. It will work too to develop communications models which other academic health centers can tailor to their own communities.

The Public Education section is also responsible for internal communication at the Supercenter, and there is an abundant amount of that. Monday is meeting day; investigators and other project personnel meet twice a month and each division once. Most people involved find, somewhat to their surprise, that they learn a great deal from the cross-fertilization of ideas that goes on at these meetings, indeed, may even enjoy them. The communicator may have to stifle an occasional yawn when the scientist starts talking about his protein synthesis, but as one community-oriented staffer put it: "I learned how lipids collect and clog the blood vessels and how my laboratory colleagues are working to solve that problem, and that has helped me understand the dimensions of my job. The opposite is true too. The hard scientists are finding out about things in the community they never even dreamed about."

The only practical result of hard and behavioral scientist togetherness thus far is the Evans-Horning collaboration which led to the saliva-nicotine test. But at least a dialogue has been opened between them. Perhaps it will help dispel the skepticism about behavioral science which is fairly common among biomedical scientists everywhere. Even Dr. DeBakey, with carefully designed smoking and diet modification studies underway in his own laboratories, joined in the chorus at a

67

National Heart and Lung Advisory Council meeting in the fall of 1975: "I don't know much about behavioral science. I don't know enough about it to know if it really is a science, and not just social studies."

Is behavioral science, science? Can it, through carefully controlled studies, produce quantifiable results and duplicable models? Can the Baylor Supercenter investigators accomplish more working together in a targeted fashion and communicating their results to the community, than they could by working by themselves, hotel fashion?

The first National Heart and Blood Vessel Research and Demonstration Center has put an elaborate evaluation plan in place to determine the anwers to such questions. Each division, indeed each project, has its short and long term goals. Each has in-house advisory committees and outside consultant-advisors. A special evaluation unit headed by a computer modeling and operations research specialist recruited from the Massachusetts Institute of Technology will monitor the whole effort, as will the National Heart and Lung Institute.

Many will be interested to see what they find out, in Houston and outside of it. The Supercenter is experimenting with a new look in health research. Considering the pressures for practical applications, its style may be a portent for the entire NIH.

5.   The Disease of the Month Club

Elbow your way off the packed elevator at the seventh floor of the Clinical Center, turn right on corridor 7 West, and say hello to Judy Lambis. She's the petite olive skinned 20 year old patient with pronounced cheek bones wearing a T-shirt which says "Kiss Me, I'm a Greek," casually chatting as she wheels about the drug transfusion she is taking from a bottle hanging off a coat hanger-like apparatus. Her older brother Nick, who has a job here on campus as a personnel clerk, drops by at lunchtime. Like several thousand people in the United States, Nick and Judy suffer from Cooley's anemia or thalassemia (named after the Detroit doctor who identified it and the Greek word sea). This means they have inherited a disease most common among people of Mediterranean descent, a serious anemia which makes it impossible for their bodies to produce red blood cells with the amount of hemoglobin usually needed to survive long past childhood; those weak cells they do produce last a few weeks, instead of the normal three or four months. Every three weeks or so they get a blood transfusion, and they have had so many that the treatment now leaves their arms sore and uncomfortable, and more importantly, leaves their bodies overloaded with iron. So the doctors give them periodic doses of the drug Desferal, which chelates or traps the iron, a drug which upsets Judy and sometimes gives her hives. They understand the limits of their treatment; they know how weak and sick they get without it;

they remember that before they came to the Clinical Center their family with its eight children used to pay hundreds of dollars every time they both went to the hospital. Judy: "The doctors here are very good doctors. They are so nice. We are getting the best treatment in the world at NIH." Nick: "We are hoping for a cure some day. Every time we ask the doctors they say they are further ahead than they were ten years ago."

The Clinical Center is a beehive; files, refrigerators, and Rube Goldberg-like equipment are piled in many corridors, and white coated scientists weave their way between them. Some say you can judge a laboratory by the amount of bustle and clutter, and if that is so, the Molecular Hematology Branch around the corner from Nick and Judy's rooms rates high. There, their chief doctor, W. French Anderson, works, well aware of his patients' hopes which are identical to his own. But he is realistic about them; he knows it may be another ten years or more before his laboratory research comes to fruition in terms of helping Cooley's victims. It was because he found himself increasingly uncomfortable with this slow pay off that he has worked to develop new chelators to remove the pathological stores of iron from his patients' blood, and thus increase their life span.

Dr. Anderson's is the elegant sort of basic science for which the National Heart and Lung Institute intramural program is renowned. For nine years now he and his colleagues have been studying the molecular basis of genetic blood disorders, patiently fractionating bone marrow cells, taking them apart infinitesimal bit by bit—first the cytoplasm, then the nucleus so they can better understand what makes them develop in the right or wrong way. "It's like a car," he explains. "You can watch an intact car run around and learn a few things. But if you really want to engineer that car, you have to take every single component apart and see what happens when you vary that component." What he and his colleagues are best known for, in the world of science, is their identification of "Human Messenger RNA," that tiny part of the cell nucleus

70

which tells the rest of the cell what to do. Now, working with human cells as well as animal models, they are pursuing several different paths: trying to find out what goes wrong when individual hemoglobin cells do not carry enough message; fusing human and rodent cells together and pulling out the individual chromosomes better to analyze the genes which make the hemoglobin; scrutinizing the bone marrow of sheep and goats to see if it might not be possible to switch off abnormal genes and to switch on normal ones such as those enjoyed during the fetal state.

Asked about a science policy matter, one of Anderson's colleagues shook his head, told of a 7 a.m.—7 p.m. working day and the stacks of scientific papers waiting his perusal, admitted he had not had the time to think about it: "The science consumes me". Anderson has been consumed to a certain degree; he and his pediatric-surgeon wife, Kathy, have intentionally not had children, because they felt their work precluded the time necessary to raise children properly. But he has had the hunch that outside forces might consume science if the scientist does not take the trouble to try to understand them. Over the years he has enrolled in several Civil Service Commission courses for federal executives and science program administrators, including courses on the federal budget, contract management, management of scientific organizations, and a legislative roundtable addressed, he recalls, by one Rep. Gerald Ford and "Mrs. Lasker's lobbyist" (Mike Gorman). Characteristically he analyzes his own motivations: "I wanted to understand how the legislative system works. I never wanted to be a one lab, one module, one technician scientist; I knew I wanted to be involved in major programs. Congress is the only place which can fund the size of the program I thought was necessary to do the work I wanted to do." Mary Lasker had understood the same thing a quarter of a century earlier.

French Anderson started at the Clinical Center on his own, with one technician. Now this Harvard, Cambridge

71

University and Harvard Medical School trained physician-scientist who has worked under Nobelists Sir Francis Crick and Dr. Marshall Nirenberg, heads a 30 person—$1.6 million laboratory (including research and patient care). He appreciates the Congressional desire to respond to the wishes of the public, including the health needs of various groups, both because the Congress wishes to try reasonably hard to meet broad social needs, and for more selfish, albeit democratic reasons ("What's a Congressman's first rule? To get reelected. What's a Congressman's second rule? To get reelected. That's one thing I learned in my Legislative Roundtable course").

As a public servant he too wants to respond to the most urgent social needs of those who foot his laboratory bills. And as a physician and human being he knows so well the hopes of patients such as Nick and Judy, that he does not mind being targeted in their direction.

But as a scientist, he understands the very basic scientists' view that they must be let go to work in ways they perceive to be most fertile because one never knows where the findings might lie. He does not think the two views are necessarily incompatible, even in a tight economy. So long as the scientists are productive, they can work within broad socially-oriented perimeters in their search for basic knowledge. The trouble is, he has seen too many turn toward the easy, the pedestrian thing as they grew older, falling into the unproductive trap of "just churning the stuff out".

To ward off such personal mediocrity he has often switched gears a bit. Last summer, he went to Cold Spring Harbor, New York, and took a crash course in cell biology so he could work at the bench a little differently. He has several times visited the sheep farm his Branch contracts with in Virginia, and one long hot day, worked there as a hired hand. Every so often he rereads John Gardner's "Self-Renewal", and after the last reading, reorganized his laboratory so he can take Wednesday afternoons to think creatively. In the past few years, he has needed many such Wednesday afternoons: For

72

into his basic laboratory of Molecular Hematology at the NHLI has fallen the prime on-campus responsibility for research concerning two vigorously targeted, emotionally tinged diseases: sickle cell disease and Cooley's anemia.

The bioscientists had hoped that their success in keeping the Heart and Lung Institute within NIH, and in themselves setting the broad priorities within the Act, boded well for them, and for the cause of basic or individually initiated research. But in the decade of the 1970s, the Congress seemed to sharpen its determination to suggest or even tell the Institutes what to study.

During the Golden Years, the House and Senate had always expressed their wishes to the NIH, the government's health research arm. This was most often done through the appropriations or funding health subcommittees, headed by those two staunch advocates of medical research, Senator Lister Hill and Congressman John Fogarty. These committees might either earmark or set aside a portion of an appropriation or increase it for a specific purpose. Or, they might simply request that the Institutes study a certain problem or emphasize it in the reports accompanying appropriations measures. The NIHers expected and accepted such directives. In fact, with the knowledgeable Dr. James Shannon at the helm, and potent supportive lobbying forces in the wings, they were known to take advantage of them, actively seeking earmarks or study requests for research they considered promising.

The appropriations directives continue, and they continue to affect NIH policies. But after the War on Cancer watershed, the authorization subcommittees, or those committees responsible for drawing up health measures and not for funding them, increasingly took the initiative.

This included, but went well beyond the traditional broad categorical approach on which the Institutes had been built: "Thou shall study Cancer," or "Thou shall study Heart

Disease", the great killers feared by millions the world over. The new thrust, or targeting, usually took a narrower form. NIH was directed to study, and thus hopefully to produce cures for ills primarily affecting certain ethnic groups, as Cooley's anemia affects those Americans of Greek or Italian descent, or as sickle cell disease affects Black people. NIH was also directed to study diseases affecting people regardless of race or ethnicity or religion, but which somehow have fallen between the institutional cracks and not commanded the attention determined and often well organized groups of public supporters—some big, some small—feel they deserve. These ranged from diabetes, an illness affecting between 4 and 5 million people, to Huntington's chorea, a neurological disorder suffered by about 14,000.

Beginning with the Cancer Act in 1971, there have been 17 Congressional initiatives which have had substantial influence on NIH programming—25 percent of all the legislation that has affected NIH since the Laboratory of Hygiene was set up in 1887 in Staten Island. The list of afflictions targeted, excluding Cancer and Heart, Lung and Blood Diseases and Arthritis (which were already targeted in their own Institutes) included:

Sickle Cell Anemia (Public Law 92-294)

Digestive Diseases (Public Law 92-305)

Cooley's Anemia (Public Law 92-414)

Multiple Sclerosis (Public Law 92-563)

Sudden Infant Death Syndrome (Public Law 93-270)

Chronic Exposure to Sulfur Oxides (Public Law 93-319)

Diabetes (Public Law 93-354)

Burns (Public Law 93-498)

Huntington's Chorea and Epilepsy (Public Law 94-63)

And there was some legislative action aiming to target Tay-Sachs, a genetic disease suffered by Jewish people. The Executive Branch usually opposes the creation of new

74

Institutes; obviously their number could not be expanded indefinitely to include every known human disorder, and in any case, setting up elaborate redundant administrative structures might further fragment and absorb health research dollars. The only completely new Institutes established in the past dozen years cover two broader than disease categories, Aging (Public Law 93-296) and Environmental Health Sciences (set up by Secretarial order). Aging, backed by well organized and sophisticated lobbies representing more than 20 million Americans over 65 could even overcome a Presidential veto to move research on growing old en masse from Child Health and Human Development to a new Institute. But even a widespread and serious disease like diabetes could not command its own Institute.

Did this mean diabetes would not be studied at NIH's busy laboratories? Obviously not. Targets are generally assigned either to a specific Institute or to the HEW for general department action. Diabetes and multiple sclerosis, for example, went to HEW commissions staffed by NIH; digestive diseases to the Arthritis Institute, along with a directive changing its name to include them. (Lobbyists insist a field moves much faster when your name is on the door.) Since the National Heart and Lung Institute under Dr. Theodore Cooper enjoyed a reputation for managerial astuteness, that Institute was handed sickle cell disease, a delicate research target tinged with racial and ethnic feelings, as well as those normally accompanying human suffering. ("We thought they could handle it," remembers a Building One official still in a position of command). Cooley's anemia went to an inter-institute committee headed by a NHLI scientist-administrator.

As the battery of directives increased, so did the appearance of the culture gap between most NIHers and their legislative masters. Those elected to serve the public by and large felt, like Connecticut's Governor (and former Representative) Ella Grasso, that "the function of government is to help meet the needs of people and health care is a prime need. Our citizens must have a voice in determining how their tax dollars

75

are used. For this reason elected representatives must be responsive to peoples' wishes in helping to set priorities for medical research and other activities supported by public funds." Many legislators also argued that tax paying constituents had received too few sure cure dividends from their now two billion dollar annual investment in NIH, and they found some support in the Nixon Administration, which, especially in the case of sickle cell, was more attuned to voter wishes than to the needs and opinions of academically oriented researchers.

Acknowledging that the more cynical among them had begun to refer to the new trend as "The Disease of the Month Club", Hill health staff and lobbyists agreed with LeRoy Goldman, staff director of the Senate Health Subcommittee, that "some distinguished members of the scientific community fall strangely silent when their own month comes along". They pointed out that Americans across the land tend to organize into voluntary groups. In health, they organize around disease entities they or their families and friends suffer, and impart their sense of urgency to the Congress—a Congress set up by the Founding Fathers to be responsive to those who knock at its doors. That is how the democratic process works. With health dollars more precious and more tightly controlled, why should not the publicly funded NIH tackle those diseases of most urgent public concern?

The NIHers perceived the matter differently. They held that Congressional enthusiasm for targeting, except in the case of cancer, was not matched with the ammunition required to hit the target. More often than not, Congress did not provide either the extra manpower or money to support its new initiatives; consequently they had to be drawn from a finite pool. For example, although it cost NIH $6,500,000 to set up six Commissions and Panels between 1972 and 1975, the Congress only provided one tenth that amount, or $650,000.

More importantly for the NIHers, the Disease of the Month Club epitomized the politicization of medical research, the irrational fragmentation of a once integrated effort, the frittering away of resources in areas with little scientific opportunity. As is so often the case, one of their number spoke for them on the editorial pages of *Science**. Pointing out that targets, or well defined clearly visualized goals, are sometimes deceptive, NIH Deputy Director for Science DeWitt Stetten Jr. wrote, "As in war, so in science one of the most difficult judgments the investigator is called upon to make is the selection of a target toward the conquest of which he will dedicate his resources".

Stetten, a former Arthritis official, General Medical Sciences Institute director and Rutgers Medical School dean, explained that maps may be inaccurate or misread, judgment of target size and distance erroneous, and estimates of ammunition needs faulty. He told a historical anecdote and drew some moral conclusions: During the War of 1812, the British Royal Navy selected the modest fishing village of St. Michaels, on Maryland's eastern shore, as a vulnerable target. Aware of their peril, the villagers agreed to extinguish every light in St. Michaels and hang lanterns from the branches of trees in a nearby forest. All night long, on August 10, 1813, the British ships lobbed cannonballs at their target, most of which fell harmlessly among the trees. The morals:

1. The identification of the proper target may be more difficult than is generally supposed.

2. Aiming at the wrong target can be enormously costly in terms of ammunition and other resources.

3. In selecting a target one should secure and study the latest and most sophisticated available information. This conclusion is equally true whether the target be military or scientific.

Leonard J. Patricelli looks back on it all somewhat incredulously. The president of WTIC television and radio station in Hartford, Connecticut, never dreamed he was starting a national war on disease when, in November of 1970,

---

Science, 19 July, 1974.

he went on the air to editorialize about a little known ailment suffered almost exclusively by Black people—50,000 of them in the United States:

> Here are some facts: There is no known cure for sickle cell anemia. There is little research being done to seek a cure. No foundation exists for the study of the disease. While volunteer groups raised nearly two million dollars for cystic fibrosis and nearly eight million for muscular dystrophy last year, less than one hundred thousand dollars was raised to combat sickle cell anemia.

In New England, birthplace of the town meeting, Patricelli thought he might excite some local interest and some action. A civic minded businessman with a long standing concern for minority problems, he had worked with Hartford's Black community in various civil rights causes. He had learned about sickle cell disease not there, but from his son Robert, then Deputy Undersecretary in the United States Department of Health, Education, and Welfare. Robert Patricelli, in turn, had learned about it from a young HEW fellow or intern, Colbert King, in the course of trying to respond to a request from the White House's John Ehrlichman to develop health options for President Nixon's upcoming programs.

King had not suffered sickle cell himself, nor had his family, but he was deeply concerned about the disease. After visits with doctors at NIH and Howard University, he reported that it is characterized by severe anemia, by bone pain and by increased susceptibility to infection; that it can cause episodes of racking pain or crises; that it is transmitted when each parent has a sickle cell gene or trait which causes blood cells to sickle or change shape, and that a million Americans carry this, in itself harmless trait. (King, now legislative assistant to Maryland's Senator Charles McC. Mathias, Jr. felt negatively about NIH after his visit there, and still thinks it is an agency prone to ivory towerism—one that says "give us the money and we'll do what we think is best").

The Patricellis, father and son, agreed with Colbert King that too little attention had been paid sickle cell and set about trying to remedy this fact. Leonard Patricelli describes the initial reaction to his efforts in the Black community as "strange." He remembers people feared there might be a stigma attached to a Black disease; they told him they had enough trouble as it was (a feeling which was magnified and complicated during the national effort later on). Still he and his colleagues persisted and gained cooperation in their campaign against sickle cell, airing editorials, announcements and news features, importing experts like Howard University's Dr. Roland B. Scott for prime-time documentaries, and raising money for a sickle cell center at Howard. The response was gratifying to say the least: The Hartford public schools started a program screening youngsters for the trait, the Connecticut state legislature began consideration of a bill providing mass screening and genetic counseling, the state medical society sponsored a symposium for medical professionals under a WTIC grant.

In Washington, Robert Patricelli too found the wheels turned unusually swiftly in response to the health option he had chosen among a field of some 140. HEW Secretary Elliot Richardson was especially sympathetic, and a Nixon Administration gearing up for the 1972 election was naturally attracted to the idea of a war on a major cause of suffering among the nation's twenty million Black citizens—an idea, what's more, which had been comparatively neglected by their Democratic predecessors. In his health message to the Congress on February 18, 1971, President Nixon targeted first cancer, and second, sickle cell anemia for concentrated research:

> It is a sad and shameful fact that the causes of this disease have been largely neglected throughout our history. We cannot rewrite this record of neglect, but we can reverse it. To this end, this administration is increasing its budget for research and treatment of sickle cell disease fivefold.

79

Connecticut's Representative Ella T. Grasso, had already inserted some WTIC editorials containing information about the tragedy of sickle cell in the Congressional Record; it would have been hard for any legislator not to vote for a war against that grim disease. The Congress hurried to overtake the Presidential initiative. A spate of bills, including one drawn up by the entire Black Caucus was introduced and the National Sickle Cell Anemia Control Act of 1972 was adopted overwhelmingly in May. It authorized a $144 million, 3 year national program for diagnosis and treatment of sickle cell disease and for counseling and research.

It was against this background that two other Connecticut residents, the late Michael Iovene and Dorothy Guiliotis, brought the disease Iovene suffered and Mrs. Guiliotis' sister had died of, to Congressional attention. Iovene, a 30 year old Ph.D. candidate in chemistry, and his friend, an officer of the modest Cooley's Anemia Blood and Research Foundation for Children's Connecticut Chapter, went to see Representative Robert N. Giaimo one wintry Saturday in his office in New Haven's Post Office Building. Sickle cell was in the air, especially in Connecticut, and the two Connecticut citizens of Mediterranean descent—he Italian, she Greek—felt they simply had to call official attention to another more serious genetic blood disease: Cooley's anemia.

It was not surprising that Congressman Giaimo had never heard of the disease, though he, and many of his constituents are of Mediterranean descent. Few people had. He listened sympathetically as his callers told him about Cooley's anemia—that it is a killer, and there is no known cure; that its victims can be identified early in life; that the only thing doctors could then do for Cooley's patients was to give them frequent blood transfusions which in turn overload the body with lethal iron. Later WTIC-TV in Hartford featured Iovene and Dorothy Guiliotis in a half hour documentary program, on which Iovene spoke poignantly, not only about his symptoms, but about how it feels to live as a Cooley's victim, dependent on the hospital and even looking different—more like his fellow Cooley's victims than his friends. (The grossly overactive bone marrow of those who suffer this disease tends to produce a thickening of the facial bones, and their slanting eyes and darker skin pigmentation gives them the oriental look Michael Iovene reported he was teased about as a child).

Back in Washington, Giaimo tried to amend the sickle cell anemia bill to include Cooley's anemia in any genetic research and screening program. When that bill was being debated on the House of Representatives floor in March, he explained his perceptions of the dimensions of this disease (200,000, he said then; experts estimated later that 5-15,000 actually suffer the disease and now that the number of Americans with transfusion-dependent Cooley's anemia, is about 2500). "I do think," Giaimo stated, "if we are going to undertake this job at long last, we should not stop on the 1 yard line—we ought to go the additional one yard and do the complete job in this area of trying to find a cure for anemia and to set up a proper screening process". And he asked a question few of his colleagues could answer negatively: "Are we going to say 'no' to the many millions who may not be afflicted but who may be carriers of Cooley's anemia, to those people whose ancestors came from the Mediterranean area, are we going to say—We are not going to do anything for your children or for you?"

But it was too late to convince the bill's floor managers to include a little known disease with the by then familiar sickle cell measure. Giaimo agreed to introduce his own bill and thus started Cooley's on what he called the orthodox route through the committee system, a route through which the Congressmen could hear expert testimony and learn more about it. The support from the small Cooley's anemia groups around the country was hardly what an American Cancer Society could muster; the opposition of the Nixon Administration during the hearings (on the grounds that it already had the authority to do the job) did not help either. Realizing their limited political assets, Mrs. Guiliotis and her fellow lobbyists enlisted the support of such ethnic groups as the Orders of Sons of Italy and AHEPA (composed of Hellenic or Greek-Americans, a fraternity which has now made Cooley's anemia a national project), and a number of northeastern lawmakers with many constituents of Mediterranean descent gave it strong support. Massachusetts' Edward Kennedy introduced the House bill in the Senate on August 9—where a similar measure had been introduced the month before by Connecticut's Senator Abraham Ribicoff—and it passed that same day. The National Cooley's Anemia Control Act followed the Sickle Cell Act into law on August 29,1972. It authorized $11.1 million for three years of research in the diagnosis and treatment of Cooley's anemia, and for counseling and public information programs.

Like the sickle cell measure, it was never explicitly funded through the appropriations process. Representative Grasso, who had become interested through WTIC's Leonard Patricelli and the WTIC documentary featuring Michael Iovene, worked with Giaimo to convince the House leadership of the need to appropriate specific dollars to accompany the Congressional mandate. To no avail; research and services for both programs were to be supported from the general health budget.

In his Clinical Center Molecular Hematology branch, Dr. W. French Anderson watched with mixed feelings as the two programs were put in place. His institute, the National Heart and Lung Institute, carved out specific funding for sickle cell when it was made the lead agency for the attack on that disease, and the NIH set up an inter-institute committee on Cooley's anemia with representatives from each institute supporting blood research, but with no extra funding.

He had no problems with the Cooley's anemia research target; far from it—Cooley's fit in precisely with the molecular studies his laboratory had undertaken; in fact, he had already recruited Nick and Judy Lambis and several other Cooley's victims as Clinical Center patients, and Dr. Arthur Nienhuis, a respected young hematologist, as the chief of clinical service.

He was pleased to see national attention focused on two cruel genetic blood diseases and became chairman of both the Cooley's HEW inter-agency and NIH inter-institute committees. The latter group moved expeditiously, setting up top priority research projects, drumming up interest in Cooley's anemia through workshops and meetings, and perhaps most immediately important, supporting—through the National Institute of Arthritis, Metabolism and Digestive Diseases—the development and preliminary testing of new iron chelators to replace the one Nick and Judy were taking.

Anderson only wished the Congress had funded its Cooley's anemia research target more clearly—that it had authorized specific funds, no matter how few, and then appropriated them, and that the funds had then been used for the specified purposes. His own laboratory was not affected; in any case he felt it had enough money, for the time being, to handle its chosen research responsibilities. Still, some of the small politically unsophisticated voluntary Cooley's anemia groups had a difficult time tolerating the lack of both new research and to a greater degree the lack of new activity on the services, information and education front under the new law. A few, such as Dorothy Guiliotis' organization, now the Connecticut Campaign Against Cooley's Anemia, came to understand that the Congress had authorized funds but appropriated no extra money for new Cooley's anemia activities. But many families, deeply concerned for their seriously sick children, and some concerned extramural scientists as well, were naturally upset when they asked what the government was doing under the new law, at being handed a list, lumping together Anderson's ongoing program ($1.6 million) and the regular NIH extramural grants research ($2.4 million). Was this the new $4 million Cooley's anemia program for which the Congress had authorized $11.1 million for a three year period?

When it came to the sickle cell target—much bigger in terms of numbers of Americans affected and support—it was a

83

different story. Cooley's victims cannot make enough red blood cells. Sickle cell victims make these cells well enough, but somehow, they go wrong; they "sickle" or change from a round shape to one resembling the tool used to cut grain or high grass. The two disease problems are different. Dean Robert Berliner of Yale Medical School, the man who, as Anderson's NHLI scientific chief, gave him the go ahead to start his laboratory, explains that medical scientists have identified the basic flaw in sickle cell disease—a defective hemoglobin which was probably the result of a gene mutation in Africa generations ago. The problem in attacking the disease stems from the paucity of ideas as to what to do about it. Many feel if the decision to target sickle cell had been made on scientific grounds alone, it never would have been made, for there were many diseases where there was much richer scientific opportunity and much more chance of progress.

On the other hand, the cause of Cooley's anemia remained a mystery and to unravel it, Dr. French Anderson believed his laboratory had to go back to study the genetic material which carries the blueprint of human life, DNA; if it proved successful, it would create a model which could then be applied in the study of other diseases. He felt, in 1972, that the sickling problem did not fit into the Molecular Hematology Branch's work, as Cooley's did. Theory aside, the instrumentation needed to study the sickling process with the necessary sophistication was not even available, and he so informed his superiors as the first $10 million and later $16 million sickle cell program got underway. In those days he got two or three calls a week, sometimes two or three a day, from government administrators, congressional staff, or physicians in Washington and elsewhere, asking him if his branch admitted sickle cell patients to the Clinical Center. No one ever told him to admit patients; requests were just that—requests. His reasons for refusing them were threefold.

The first was a matter of principle. Anderson's was a research laboratory; it did work important to scientific

84

research. It would admit perhaps 20 or 25 patients if there were good reasons scientifically; if there were no such reasons, it would not admit the patients "to make Richard Nixon or anyone else look good politically." Had he not been so adamant, Anderson recalls, he could have gotten a lot of people in the Administration off the hook by admitting a number of prominent Black people with sickle cell disease: "Then the Administration would have been able to say: 'Look at what we are doing for the sickle cell effort: the Mayor's aunt is at NIH.' " It would have given the appearance of progress toward a solution, when there was no such solution in sight.

The second reason was a scientific one. Anderson did not think he could scientifically justify dropping the long range approach his laboratory was using—an approach he still thinks will ultimately provide the answers for genetic blood disorders—"to do short term work to satisfy politicians." He respected the point of view of these politicians, and understood they were just trying to do their jobs as he tried to do his. If there were anything he could really have done for sickle cell patients, that would have been one thing. But there was nothing he could do except prescribe such old-fashioned remedies as bed rest and healthy nutrition, and in the case of very sick patients, the kind of care available in any community hospital.

Anderson felt what ideas there were could be tried out in other places, especially through the various Institute extramural grant programs. This in fact, did occur; enough research on the subject had accumulated by 1974 to permit NHLI to hold a national symposium where investigators described their efforts. There has been no quick research payoff. Two ideas which at first excited a lot of hoopla did not prove out too successfully: treatment of sickle cell disease through the use of the chemical compounds urea (ineffective) and cyanate (still some question as to its effect, especially if the patient's blood is processed outside the body, but it causes notable side effects in a few patients when taken by mouth).

French Anderson had a third reason. He felt that a key, though usually unstated motive of the sickle cell program would be frustrated if he began to use sickle cell monies in his well established intramural laboratory. He believed the Black scientific community to be caught in a vicious cycle: the Black universities and scientific groups often could not compete successfully for NIH grant monies unless they were reasonably productive, and they could not become reasonably productive unless they could compete successfully for grant monies. Why not now give these medical scientists their fair chance under the new sickle cell program?

The consensus is that most did get the chance. And though a considerable number of NIHers criticized the use of NHLI research funds to support a largely service program, they agreed that real progress was made for patients in terms of health, education and thoughtful, compassionate care. The sickle cell program reached people who had never enjoyed such care or had ready access to information about such subjects as proper nutrition. But it had to weave its way through a maze of racial sensitivities as the Department of Health, Education, and Welfare established 24 sickle cell screening and education clinics across the country (funded by NHLI and administered by the Health Services Administration) and NHLI set up 15 comprehensive sickle cell centers in academic medical centers, combining research with community education, screening and diagnosis.

Many in the Black community feared the new emphasis on a Black disease, as Leonard Patricelli had discovered in Hartford in the beginning. They were proved right, to some degree. All the publicity generated a great deal of questionable, if well intentioned, activity: a few states enacted compulsory sickle cell screening laws and many well meaning voluntary groups jumped on the bandwagon to sponsor screening without the proper medical follow-up or counseling. It took years to iron out the initial confusion between people identified in hastily set up inexpert screening programs, as carriers having the sickle cell trait, and those actually suffering the disease; meanwhile, many with the trait could not get jobs or were refused insurance or admission to educational institutions. Even at NIH itself a screening program had to be cancelled when protesting Black employees felt the data gathered could be put in their work files and misused. Most experts now feel that public education must precede actual screening activities, be they voluntary or involuntary, or great personal suffering can result. In fact, Cooley's voluntary groups later agreed, in light of the sickle cell experience, that small pilot research studies on screening and counseling methods would be far preferable to mass screening. ("What should we do?" asked one involved in the effort, "take a truck down to the Italian neighborhood and scare everyone by announcing we are screening for Cooley's anemia?")

What's more, the genetic counseling which was an integral part of the new sickle cell program was a touchy business, as is any public activity which touches private lives. Some extremists objected, and even called the sickle cell effort "genocide," though couples advised about their chances of having a child with the disease if both carried the trait (1 in 4) were quite free to make their own decisions about whether to marry or have children. Misguided or not, this argument damaged even properly set up programs.

Finally, some questioned whether this early target was the right one for the Black community. Meeting at Meharry Medical College in Nashville in December of 1971, several prominent Black physician-participants in the Congressional Black Caucus-sponsored Conference on the Status of Health in the Black Community pointed out an ironic fact: though hypertension is a quieter killer than sickle cell, it affects many more people and appears three times more frequently among Blacks than Whites. And, in most cases, it is treatable.

The years passed. NIH Building One officials feel it their function to protect intramural scientists, to act as buffers

87

between them and the political powers downtown. Dr. W. French Anderson's superiors backed him up; the NHLI Molecular Hematology Branch admitted occasional sickle cell patients, but no large number, to its Clinical Center beds and outpatient clinic. Then what the medical scientists call the state of the art began to change. Together with an Italian laboratory, the Heart and Lung Institute developed a new instrument which can measure the oxygen-carrying capacity of human blood cells as they actually exist in the body. Since sickling occurs under conditions of reduced oxygen, the instrument permitted the scientists to observe and study the sickling process.

Anderson and Nienhuis recruited The Johns Hopkins University's Dr. Robert Winslow, a research clinician with a major interest in sickle cell. A bit later, Dr. Rudolph Jackson, the physician who had served on the HEW Secretary's original Sickle Cell Advisory Board and headed up the extramural NIH program, joined the laboratory's staff. Thus equipped, the Branch began in 1975 to admit between 20 and 25 patients, not, as Dr. Jackson puts it, to test any particular therapeutic approach (there still was little promising to test), but to study the sickling process with the new instrument. It also aimed to assemble and computerize facts about the effects of the disease, such as the extent of organ damage in individual patients, so that doctors elsewhere will be able to learn more about what to expect of it.

On Capitol Hill, some lawmakers at least began to reconsider the Disease of the Month Club. As a result of the lobbying efforts of the genetic scientific community, especially the National Genetics Foundation, many of them became convinced that since there may turn out to be hundreds of different genetic diseases—including to some extent those which run in families like diabetes and breast cancer—there are strong medical reasons for an overall rather than a categorical approach to genetic diseases. Non-categorical genetic disease measures were introduced in both House and Senate. These aimed to repeal existing categorical authorities for diseases like

88

sickle cell and Cooley's anemia, and to replace them with broad authorities for research and services in genetic diseases. What practical effect they would have is not clear, except that they would combine the administration for genetic diseases and place it in a central place in the HEW bureaucracy. Such a law would not affect Dr. Anderson and his laboratory, or similar extramural research scientists. But it would emphasize the generic nature of genetic disease and combine the programs under one authority. Thus, it would symbolically put the brakes on targeted disease attacks.

Two Senators moved in 1975 to challenge the imbalance caused by political targeting. During the debate on the annual Department of Health, Education, and Welfare appropriation, the Senator who had cast the lone vote against the Senate Cancer bill in 1971, Gaylord Nelson of Wisconsin, introduced an amendment with Senator Alan Cranston of California. They suggested that $100 million be cut from the Cancer budget, $50 million from the Heart budget, and that $50 million of the $150 million thus saved should be redistributed among the other less favored institutes.

A strange ploy? To no one except the political novice. The Senators held out a budget-trimming carrot to the fiscal conservatives, while calling attention to what they felt was an imbalance among the institutes and a lack of emphasis on non-targeted research. They held that, even adjusting the dollars for inflation, Cancer Institute funds had grown by 186 percent between 1970 and 1975 and Heart by 52 percent, while those of the other Institutes dropped 13 percent. In the present fiscal year, they said, the total portion of NIH appropriations devoted to Cancer and Heart had risen from 31 percent in 1970 to 51 percent in 1975. Detailing examples of research approved through the peer review process but unable to be funded in such Institutes as General Medical Sciences, and Neurology, they argued this rise had been at their expense. (It was not entirely fair, as we will see, to lump Cancer and Heart together in these comparisons since Heart in these years had become Lung and Blood as well.)

Responding, Senator Edward Kennedy put on the record a report to the President from Cancer Panel Chairman Benno Schmidt which included a paean by one who, as some observed, had "really gotten religion", in support of basic research, as well as the assurance that the Cancer Institute was devoting over half its resources to its cause. He acknowledged that "we do not have in cancer the fundamental science base that was present in both the Manhattan Project and the Space program, and that is the reason that the largest area of expenditure in the Cancer Program is fundamental research designed to broaden this science base." Before other less political forums Schmidt has argued that if federal dollars had not been allocated to Cancer, they would not have gone to health research at all, and, pointed out that NCI was lending support ($16 million in 1975) to other "less fortunate" institutes for various purposes related to its own.

But it was Appropriations Subcommittee Chairman Warren Magnuson who led the counterattack and spoke for the advocates of targeting through the democratic political process. Heart disease and cancer, the Senator from Washington pointed out, account for 71 percent of the deaths in the United States, and that is why their budgets had been raised. This was a bill to meet human needs; it would be unconscionable to trade off one institute against another:

"Believe me, 20 million people in the United States who have been affected either directly or indirectly care about cancer. And if we could poll the American people right now, and ask them, 'What headline would you like to see in your morning paper when you wake up tomorrow?' most or all of them would answer four words: 'Cure for Cancer Found.' "

The Nelson-Cranston amendment was rejected 62-19. Senator Nelson had gained only 18 votes in four years, and a goodly portion of those were not votes against targeting, but conservative statements for NIH budget cutting.

When it came to minor genetic diseases affecting fractions of the population, however politically potent, Congress seemed ready to tailor its approach and go along with the latest and most sophisticated bioscientific, rather than political judgments setting medical research targets. But when it came to the great killers, especially to cancer—that evil cause of human suffering—that was a different story.

6.   The Budget Squeeze

*"Approved but not funded." What do those four words
from the bureaucratic lexicon mean? To Dr. Maria I. New, a
recognized authority on childhood hypertension, they meant a
serious, year long slowdown in the search for new knowledge.
Head of the Division of Pediatric Endocrinology and
Professor of Pediatrics at New York Hospital-Cornell Medical
Center, she had a grant from the National Heart and Lung
Institute over a period of a half dozen years — a grant rising
from about $12,500 in 1969 ($10,000 to her research work, the
rest in indirect overhead costs to her institution) to more than
$21,500 in 1973 ($13,700 in direct costs, the rest to her
institution), to investigate the exact hormonal causes of
childhood hypertension. She thinks her work is important
because though hypertension is usually treatable, physicians
do not know the cause in most patients and she was on her way
to identifying specific causes and developing recommendations
as to which drugs could be most effectively used for which
disorders. Evidently her peers — the country's leading experts
in her field — agreed; she was advised they reviewed her
application "very favorably," but that there was not enough
money to fund it. For a while a sense of panic seized her small
laboratory, jobs were placed in jeopardy and she had to let one
of her two trained technicians go. Work slowed as the grant
was phased out and she wrote grant proposals seeking
alternative support.*

93

Dr. New's curriculum vitae runs for nine pages, detailing a substantial list of research and hospital appointments as well as an impressive scientific bibliography. Her name was known well enough to enable her to piece together support from several sources as she reapplied to the NHLI and received a grant of $52,000 to continue her work ($32,000 in direct costs, the rest in indirect costs. The size of an average annual individual grant has now risen from about $35,000 to $55,000.) In the same way, Dr. Daniel Deykin, a Professor at Tufts and Boston University School of Medicine was able to continue part of his series of studies of the regulatory mechanisms of blood clotting under a smaller substitute Veterans' Administration grant when his application for a large $372,000 program project grant (about $286,000 for research, the rest to his institution in indirect or overhead costs) to continue support of a 30-40 person laboratory was "approved but not funded" by NHLI. But it took time to reapply and he had to let people go and drop projects which might have proved important, including an examination in patients with leukemia of the tiny blood cells, or platelets, which play a critical part in starting blood clotting and an investigation of the role of platelets and blood clotting in patients with coronary heart disease.

To another very established investigator, Dr. William Insull Jr. of Rockefeller University, the loss of his "approved but not funded" NHLI grant meant a loss of pace and time too. But it meant more. It meant that in scrounging about for support for his basic research on lipid metabolism — how body fats interact with the cells of the artery walls to cause arteriosclerosis — he has had to tailor an innovative approach to make it more attractive to industrial funding sources. An old peer reviewer himself, he is sympathetic to the notion that perhaps there was some fat on the NIH-university research establishment's bones a decade ago. Yet now, he says, "not only have they cut the fat, they are beginning to get the meat on the bones." He explains that such funding cuts have secondary

94

implications less noticeable but perhaps more significant than the effect on individual laboratories. Most importantly, there has been a slippage that tends to impair the quality of research as investigators like himself are forced to abandon their basic step by step climb up the wall of knowledge to attempt a swift leap up to practical applications. Quality slips; the safe vogue thing gets higher priority than risky speculative research. In his case, he feels his present pharmaceutical industry supported investigation of fat-lowering drugs to be less powerful than the job he could have done had he had more time to develop more basic knowledge about body fat metabolism.

Across the country, at the University of Southern California School of Medicine's Shock Research Unit, Dr. Max Harry Weil has also had to reduce his commitment to the sort of quality clinical research he wanted to do. He had headed a large medical and non-medical group investigating the shock which follows heart attack and possible treatment for it — how the body reacts to this catastrophic insult and what mechanical and electronic devices might be developed to monitor its reactions and give doctors the ability to respond promptly and efficiently. Since his application to NHLI to continue that work was "approved but not funded" that group has been cut in half and he has proceeded with support pieced together from a private foundation and other smaller Public Health Service grants. "Is our research alive?" asks Dr. Weil. "Some is, and some is not. Are we capable of being as productive as we were? No, we are not."

To the young investigators, those under 40 who have not had time to compile extensive bibliographies and lists of committees and appointments, the words "approved but not funded" can have a more devastating meaning. Had 31 year old Dr. Richard L. Coulson's grant application to NHLI been funded as well as approved, he would have been well on his way as an independent investigator. He and his seniors at Temple University Medical School's Laboratory of Cardiology in Philadelphia had high hopes for his first application. As a

95

research associate at University College in London he had developed a technique using an old drug — nitroglycerine — for a new purpose: elucidating the performance of skeletal muscle. Now, as a full time Temple University researcher, he wanted to use the same technique to measure the performance of that most important muscle, the heart, in animals; his ultimate aim was to discover what particular aspects of metabolism are deranged during congestive heart failure. He was determined, and so were his superiors; they managed to piece together some support for a year while he begged, borrowed and scavenged equipment. He describes himself as not discouraged, but disappointed and puzzled; he had counted on a future in cardiovascular research, a field which he feels has not reached its full potential and which is crucial for the health of millions of Americans.

"What do you do with what you are sure is a good research idea when you cannot get it funded?" asks Richard Coulson. "That is the riddle." Dr. Peter H. Levine is trying to solve a similar riddle. This 37 year old Director of the Hemophilia Center and Blood Coagulation Laboratory at the Memorial Hospital in Worcester, Massachusetts, works in the field of hemophilia, the inherited bleeding disorder associated with the sons of czars and kings, but suffered by some 25,000 commoners in the United States. Dr. Levine, a professor of medicine at the University of Massachusetts, has developed a self-therapy protocol for hemophiliacs—a recipe under which patients, with their families' help, can treat themselves before the onset of physical symptoms. When his grant application to NHLI to test this new methodology on a larger scale, using new clotting agents or drugs, was "approved but not funded," he was not personally upset: "No one is. There just isn't enough money to go around." But he pointed out the government may have been penny wise and pound foolish: now huge amounts of money are spent treating hemophiliac patients in emergency rooms after the fact; smaller tests have shown his self therapy program could bring costs down by about 40 percent.

Happily, says Dr. Levine, he is a good enough teacher so that the loss of the usual status enjoyed by a funded investigator in the academic pecking order has made little difference to him, careerwise. Still, he is anxious: another smaller research grant application has been "approved but not funded" by NHLI — this one to investigate a new phenomenon, how white blood cells inhibit the way platelets work on blood vessel walls. He cannot continue to spend two or three weeks to prepare a proposal the size of a small telephone book only to have it "approved but not funded" and he has opted to do his research as part of a larger contract with ten hospitals. But it is the kind of directed research he feels is far less productive than that accomplished when an individual investigator is left free to pursue his own leads.

When Senators Gaylord Nelson and Alan Cranston argued, in the fall of 1975, for a more even distribution of funds among the National Institutes of Health, they lumped the Cancer and Heart Institutes together as recipients of disproportionately large shares.

This was not quite fair, as the cardiovascular NIHers pointed out the following December. In a belated letter to the two Senators endorsed by the entire membership of the National Heart and Lung Advisory Council, four of its members, led by the Harvard Medical School's distinguished cardiologist and Hersey Professor of Medicine, Dr. Eugene Braunwald, explained that:

> During fiscal 1967, the National Heart Institute received 15 percent and the National Cancer Institute 16 percent of all NIH research monies; five years later the National Heart and Lung Institute budget had risen to only 16 percent while the Cancer Institute budget had risen to 26 percent;

> Although the National Heart, Blood Vessel, Lung and Blood Act was passed in 1972, "the expectations for stepping up research in these vital areas were not realized"; the fraction of NIH support going to NHLI remained at 16 percent, while Cancer's rose to 34 percent;

Particularly disturbing when cardiovascular disease continues to be the primary health problem in the United States (costing the nation some $40 billion a year) was the Senators' perception that heart research had grown too rapidly at the expense of other fields; in fact, the percentage of the NIH budget devoted to research on heart and blood vessels had declined from 11 to nine percent between 1972 and 1975.

In less bureaucratic language, the job of the Institute had been expanded to cover new fields, like lung disease and blood resources, and such new activities as health education. It had also been directed by Congress to attack several diseases of the month and by formal cooperative agreements signed in 1972 and 1974, to serve as U.S. leader in an international effort in which American and Soviet scientists collaborate to study cardiovascular disease, blood transfusion, and artificial heart research.

Although its budget admittedly had increased dramatically, it had increased far less than was projected in 1972 and no extra monies had been added to cover such explicit tasks as the highly visible $16 million sickle cell disease program. Also, although the Institute's dollars had almost doubled, its staff had only increased about 13 percent.

The search for knowledge can be thought of as a continuum or a giant wheel which is accomplishing something. Each spoke has its job, each has its advocates who feel theirs is the most important spoke on the research wheel. Can you, if you have the resources, pick out just one to strengthen? Conversely, can you pick one to weaken if your resources shrink?

The basic research spoke remains totally important. If you destroy the acquisition of fundamental information which is the basis for all preventive measures, and all cures, the wheel collapses. About half of the NHLI budget goes into this search for fundamental knowledge.

But what about those scientists who take basic concepts and find or suggest new ways to apply them? If you detract from their targeted efforts, if you stop supporting clinical investigations and clinical trials which test new drugs or new surgical procedures, you have a plethora of basic facts without knowing exactly what to do with them. Though it is difficult to say precisely how much of the total NHLI budget goes into basic, and how much into applied research, clearly a fourth of the Institute's budget is now spent each year on contracts largely supporting clinical trials. Their advocates claim that such trials testing various hypotheses about the applications of new knowledge give us our best chance for preventing coronary heart disease. It is from such trials that NHLI leaders hope to get definitive information about whether the various factors apparently affecting the incidence of heart disease can, in fact, be controlled. Such testing and evaluation of existing knowledge comprises the second spoke on the research wheel.

Finally, there is the third spoke on the wheel, the translation of research results for the nation's physicians and their patients. If you do not make sure that tested research results move expeditiously from bench to bedside, and are actually used to improve health and well being, what do you have? An ivory tower program. Although finding out what causes disease surely produces the most certain way of preventing it, you cannot stick your head in the ground and ignore suffering patients while you put all your money and effort into plumbing root causes. You must apply tested research results through demonstration and education programs to "control" disease. Such activities absorb less than five percent of the NHLI budget.

The Institutes use various instruments to close knowledge gaps, take advantage of new leads, and support the search for new knowledge. Like other top NIH men,* NHLI Director

---

*Though NIH now has one woman Institute director, Dr. Ruth Kirschstein of the National Institute of General Medical Sciences, there are few women in top NIH administrative positions as in all the medical establishment.

Robert I. Levy is less concerned about the instrument of support used in any research endeavor than are some research scientists. He feels the instrument must be tailored to the search at hand. The contract mechanism is obviously more appropriate for the administration of a large scale clinical trial with a common protocol or set of procedures taking place in many different medical centers around the country than is a research grant to an individual, or even a larger program project grant to a group of investigators at one medical center. Over 25 percent of the Institute budget is now spent through contracts.

But many investigators deplore the increased use of what they feel to be targeted, clearly controlled NIH contracts, not funneled through study section-Advisory Council dual peer review system and often going to industry rather than the academic medical community. Levy responds that although NHLI contracts are not reviewed by the Institute Advisory Council, they are subject to a primary technical review by outside experts, and that over 80 percent of the Heart and Lung Institute contracts are with medical schools and universities. (The National Cancer Institute gave the contract mechanism its questionable reputation among scientists; in its cancer chemotherapy program NCI has screened thousands of drug compounds to see if they could inhibit malignancies and developed new compounds to be tested through contractual arrangements with large drug companies. And, in the Nixon years, the Institute began to operate laboratories developed by the Army at Fort Detrick, Maryland, under contract to a Litton Industries subsidiary.)

NHLI employs another targeted instrument of support, the SCOR or Specialized Center of Research, when it decides there is a need for a multi-disciplined attack on a disease. The 48 SCORs enlist pharmacologists, pathologists, histologists, biochemists, physiologists and other bioscientists in concentrated attacks on arteriosclerosis (13), hypertension (5), ischemic heart disease, or coronary heart disease (9), pulmonary diseases (17) and thrombosis or blood clotting (4). The project ideas within the SCORs come from the investigators, but the Institute defines the overall frame of reference, and in exchange for five year funding the SCORs agree to be closely monitored by SCOR-keepers to exchange information with their counterparts and even to change in midstream when that seems warranted.

In the National Research and Demonstration Centers, or supercenters, the Institute has gone a step further and asked educators, communicators and others to join scientists in targeted attacks against disease which covers the whole spectrum of research — from laboratory investigation to demonstration and education projects. It gives these supercenters long range funding and closely monitors them, as it does the SCORs. But there are as yet only three, one each in heart and blood vessel, lung and blood research. We have had a glimpse of the supercenter at Houston earlier.

The SCORs and supercenters are a bit more popular in the bioscientific community than are the contracts: the researchers have more to say about their individual design, and ongoing management. Still, such wholesale grants have their detractors who feel they milk funds which would otherwise go to individual investigators, that they are simply catch-alls for an array of university projects in search of federal funds which do not have to pass through the same stringent peer review system as do the individual grants, and that, like contracts, they reflect a desire on the part of Institute, or perhaps Administration officials, to gain control over research programming. Whether this is true, or whether, as the Congress—and indeed the bioscientific authors of the Arteriosclerosis Report which so influenced the National Heart, Blood Vessel, Lung and Blood Act—clearly felt, the time-honored system of project applications and grants had failed to explore all possible research leads, is a matter for conjecture.

In any case, the Heart and Lung Institute now attaches many more strings to its research funding than it did during the

Golden Years, when the great bulk of its funds simply provided the fire to heat up Marshall Nirenberg's "boiling soup" of thousands of individual investigators each pursuing his own idea. Mission-oriented research including contracts, SCORS, supercenters and sickle cell centers, now comprise almost 40 percent of the Institute's budget. One of the Institute's administrators expressed the new approach: "Society has a perfect right to say, 'to hell with you, buddy', to the guy who says, 'I'm a competent scientist, you owe me a technician, 3,000 feet of space and a refrigerated ultracentrifuge!' "

If the Institute cup still ran over, as it did during the Golden Years, if there were enough funds steadily to strengthen all the spokes of the research wheel, the advocates of each approach could have few complaints, and the NHLI leadership would have few problems. But in the mid-1970s, this was not the case.

The Congress had asked the Institute, in the National Heart, Blood Vessel, Lung and Blood Act of 1972, to prepare a five year plan and authorized it to spend about $535 million a year by 1975 to carry it out. But tighter budgeting had left it with only $325 million—a roughly $200 million money gap. That cold winter, it looked as though the Institute's authorization for the following year might, for the first time, sink below its current appropriation.

The five year plan, as we have seen, set three goals, the acquisition of fundamental knowledge, the testing and evaluation of existing knowledge, and the application of existing knowledge. The first, already well underway, was the traditional Institute role. It was necessary to gear up for the second, and to start the third from the beginning. Not surprisingly, the Institute turned most enthusiastically to the second goal in 1972 and 1973, when it seemed as though its budget would rise to cover many new ventures. It had had some experience with clinical trials; two were already in the pipeline. And they did not seem as alien to trained medical researchers as did public education and demonstration programming.

Some 50,000 Americans are involved in the National Heart and Lung Institute's five major trials.* Many more thousands of people have been screened for these trials under contracts with 70 medical centers around the country, and in Canada. Four of them aim in different ways to determine whether or not people can voluntarily decrease the risk of falling prey to heart disease:

LRC, the lipid research primary prevention trial, aims to test the hypothesis that lowering blood cholesterol prevents or delays heart attacks;

HDFP, the hypertension detection and follow-up program, seeks to determine if the morbidity (the amount of disease suffered) and mortality (the death rate) can be reduced in the general population by systematic anti-hypertensive drug management;

AMIS, the Aspirin Myocardial Infarction trial, tests whether giving small daily doses of aspirin helps patients who have suffered at least one heart attack;

MRFIT, or, as some call it, Mr. Fit, the Multiple Risk Factor Intervention Trial asks whether active intervention in the treatment of people who smoke, or have high blood pressure, or high blood cholesterol levels will lower their morbidity and mortality rates.

The fifth trial, CAST (the Coronary Artery Surgery Trial), will seek to ascertain whether the coronary bypass operation performed routinely by such surgeons as Dr. Michael DeBakey today, does more than alleviate pain; whether, in fact, it has an effect on the amount of disease patients suffer and the length of their lives. All the trials maintain control groups, and subjects are chosen randomly. LRC and AMIS employ a strict "double blind design." This means that neither the doctor nor the patient knows who is being treated or who is getting a placebo. CAST and AMIS are secondary prevention trials, admitting subjects who have

*The National Institutes of Health now conduct some 1100 major and minor trials.

103

already suffered disease or its symptoms, while Mr. Fit and LRC are primary prevention trials, admitting people without evidence of disease; HDFP admits both.

Now doctors have good evidence from many studies, including the Institute's well-known epidemiological study in Framingham, Massachusetts, which has followed two generations through the years, that if Americans smoke cigarettes they are more likely, and if they stop smoking cigarettes, less likely, to become heart attack victims. Doctors also know that if their patients' blood pressure and blood cholesterol levels are high, these patients run a greater risk of suffering heart disease and death. But would Americans suffer fewer first heart attacks and less killing cardiovascular disease if doctors intervened to persuade them to stop smoking and to bring their blood pressure and high cholesterol levels down, through drugs and low-fat diets?

Through MRFIT, or Mr. Fit, the NHLI hopes, within a decade, to produce the answer with scientific certainty. Because it takes less time and money to study the people most likely to have heart attacks, Mr. Fit, one of the largest and most difficult trials on an important contemporary health problem ever undertaken, has screened over 400,000 men between the ages of 35 and 57, to find the upper tenth of the population most at risk. (Experts estimate a national diet study would involve 100,000 people and cost as much as $1 billion, or much more than the total annual Institute budget.) Twelve thousand men who have at least one of the three risk factors will participate in Mr. Fit, and each will be studied for six years. Participants are to be divided at random into two groups. Half will be referred to their personal physicians for whatever care they choose, the other group will enter a special program, wherein Institute funded clinicians will try to intervene positively to help them change pleasurable ways: to stop smoking, to reduce their blood cholesterol concentrations by dieting, and to bring their blood pressure down by losing weight and taking drugs.

Mr. Fit and similar trials hold little intellectual innovative appeal for scientists who want to study the unknown, not test the known. Such NIHers hold that you do not need the high scientific competency which is the hallmark of a National Heart and Lung Institute to conduct a clinical trial, and if NIH did not support such trials, someone else would. A few Nader-like critics view the trials as a dilatory tactic, designed to delay potent government pronouncements which affect important segments of the economy. ("The dairy and egg people are afraid of this cholesterol business, they say look what all that lung cancer talk did to the cigarette industry.") Others hold the word *delay* is too dramatic; NHLI simply does not give top priority to the need to know of people who live today and eat today because it acts cautiously in the face of powerful groups who overreact before the fact to any government action. In any case, a Federal Trade Commission judge did not need to wait for the results of the NHLI elaborate clinical trials to find, in December of 1975, sufficient scientific evidence to say that the egg industry had engaged in false, misleading and deceptive advertising by claiming that eating eggs does not increase the chance of heart attacks.

Some now feel it was perhaps a mistake to start the trials in the first place. Once an Institute begins to pour money into clinical trials involving great amounts of increasingly expensive patient treatment, it has created what is in fact a budget-eating monster. Once such programs are underway, once they have begun to screen, treat and follow up significant portions of the population, they cannot be turned off. Not only would the Institute lose the huge investment it had already made but it would violate its commitment to serve thousands of participants.

"It would be a sin not to do these trials," says NHLI Deputy Director Robert Ringler, and most of his colleagues agree that at least it would be imprudent not to do them, though they take so many years and their cost now runs between $40 and $60 million a year, and threatens to escalate daily along with all costs involving medical care and treatment. Clinical trial proponents argue this is a small investment compared to the some $40 billion cardiovascular diseases now cost the nation every year. What's more, if you neglect this step and do not take the time and make the effort thoroughly to test scientific findings, you run the risk of permitting ineffective or even harmful medicines and medical procedures and practices to find their way into the health care system.

Some examples:

For years the clinically minded health lobbyists such as the Lasker forces had pushed the testing of new drugs, in the field of heart disease as well as in cancer and in mental illness. NHLI's Coronary Drug trials, launched in the mid-1960s asked this question: Do those drugs that reduce levels of certain fatty substances in the blood of men who have had at least one heart attack improve their chances of avoiding more, and living longer lives? After a six year study involving over 8,300 coronary patients, 53 participating clinics and five treatment regimes, the Institute was able to answer: "Apparently not." Indeed, three of the treatment regimes (including high and low dose estrogens) were dropped during the study when it became apparent that not only were they doing no good, but that they might be doing some harm .

In the same way, clinical trials, some supported by the Institute, have now shown that there are very few indications for the use of the anti-coagulant drugs which used to be used routinely for heart attack victims. And the cardiovascular community was sensitized to the need for the Coronary Artery Surgery Trial (CAST) now being carried out in 13 hospitals, after a trial in Seattle indicated that a similar operation rerouting the internal mammary artery, which normally supplies blood to the chest wall, to the heart, did not significantly improve patients' chances of living longer, disease free lives. About 40,000 coronary by-pass operations are performed each year in the United States at an estimated total cost of $400 million; CAST is designed to demonstrate the extent of their therapeutic effect.

So the clinical trials continue, costing ever larger sums of money, and squeezing traditional basic research at one end of the research continuum, and the new demonstration and education programs at the other. At the same time, the Congress is pushing all of the Institutes along the research continuum. It tells the government's health research agency not only to acquire and test new knowledge but to translate those findings which test out well and demonstrate them in selected parts of the population, and then to try to reach out to educate physicians and other medical workers and their patients as to their use.

A typical scenario: In a 1974 report, Senator Warren Magnuson's Appropriations Subcommittee, "completely disappointed" with NIH's response to its request for more information dissemination, asked the agency to submit a complete action report with recommendations and a plan for implementation for such information. The following year, the committee reported that NIH had submitted an acceptable statement of NIH responsibility and a reasonable plan for carrying it out. Although it agreed with NIH that unnecessary duplication of effort would be wasteful and other agencies in the federal and local governments and the private sector should join in the effort, it held "there seems to be a present danger that too little rather than too much will be done." Accordingly, the Committee looked to NIH "to assure itself that others are, in fact, adequately performing those parts of the communications task which for jurisdictional reasons, it does not propose to undertake itself."

"The Committee looks to NIH." The Congress has been hard on the Institutes in many ways, but it keeps giving them more and more jobs to do. At the National Heart and Lung Institute, Director Robert Levy points unhappily to the five volume, five year plan, and refers to the fact that though the Congress and the Plan suggested that the Institute set up 30 Research and Demonstration centers covering the whole broad spectrum of research, budget restrictions had limited it to three: "What a joke! We developed noble plans, we

107

announced competitions, attracted grant applications and aroused expectations. Then we could not really produce. It's no wonder our credibility is questioned."

NHLI had to divert $2.3 million from its traditional research grant budget to start a hypertension education program in 1972. Under HEW Secretary Elliot Richardson's leadership, it launched a nationwide effort to reach the nearly half of the 23 million Americans who did not know they suffered from the disease as well as about eight million hypertensives who knew they had it but did not have their illness properly controlled. This was apparently money well spent, for at the end of 1975 the Institute held a press conference to announce that hypertension's days as a silent killer were on the wane. Since 1971 there had been a sharp decrease in the number of Americans unaware that their blood pressure is high and a doubling of the number whose disease is under effective control. But there were still large numbers of people who were aware of their hypertension, but ignoring it or not controlling it.

The Institute now spends about $15 million on this and similar demonstration and education programs to "control" disease including the anti-smoking and fire department emergency ambulance projects underway at Dr. Michael DeBakey's supercenter at Houston, Texas, and experimental mass media campaigns in three small California towns conducted by the Stanford Heart Disease Prevention program. These campaigns seem to be effective—especially when face to face instruction or printed booklets reinforce a television or radio spot, or billboard advertisement. Their message: stop smoking, eat more wisely and exercise more and so reduce your risk of suffering a heart attack.

Such programs do not attempt to treat or educate great numbers of people. Rather, as small, carefully evaluated projects, they ask, does such and such a project work? If so, how does it work? And why? When it has answers to such questions, the Institute feels it will have produced some new approaches for many communities to try.

Some medical scientists show even less enthusiasm for the new "control" activities than for the clinical trials, and argue that the Institute strictly confine its activities in this field to advising and consulting with other agencies. Arguing that Congressmen elected every few years naturally are more attuned to immediate than long range needs (but that "the postponement of gratification is a sign of maturity") Dr. Eugene Braunwald insists that NHLI responsibilities for medical services are assumed at the expense of its traditional research grant program. "It's like inviting a starving man into your home," Braunwald, himself once a NHLI intramural investigator renowned for his research on heart disease and heart catheterization, explains. "Once you invite him in you are morally and probably legally obliged to feed him even though your own children do not have enough food. Although you have to be considerate, you cannot adopt him, or you will ruin what you have."

Whether or not the Institute's traditional research grant program now consuming almost half its $325 million budget can be likened to a threatened child depends on your point of view. But there is no doubt that this research program, which has a long standing reputation for excellence, has been caught in a budget squeeze. Peer reviewers rate grant applications on a sliding scale; 100 equals A-plus; 500, D-minus. Policy makers worry not about the few basic researchers whose grant applications are given a top 100 rating by their peers, or about those whose applications are rated 499. But what about those whose applications are judged somewhere in the middle? Might there be a prospective Madame Curie, a Jonas Salk, an Alexander Fleming among them?

Heart and Lung bureaucrats call the top rating they are able to fund the "payline" for that year. In 1967 the Heart Institute's payline hovered around 380 or more; now it is only about 220. This means though the number of Institute research dollars has increased, the proportion of grants approved by peer reviewers and recommended by the Advisory Council which have actually been funded has dropped alarmingly. In 1967, the Institute funded 90 percent of its approved grant applications, in 1975 that proportion had dropped to 52 percent. Add to this the fact that other Institutes have less favorable budgets than NHLI and the financial realities of the mid-1970s, and you begin to appreciate the fears of the bioscientific research community. Medical research has always been expensive, now it simply costs more than it used to. A study made in the NIH Director's office shows that the biomedical research price index rose 61.7 percent between 1961 and 1974 while the more general consumer price index rose only 43.8 percent. After all, laboratories are more elaborate than they used to be, equipment and drugs more complex and expensive, salaries even higher. One Institute scientific director estimates that in the seven years of his service ending this year, the cost of putting a man or woman in the laboratory went from $15,000 to $36,000.

Moreover, NHLI officials estimate that between 20 and 40 percent of what the Congress and the public regards as the "new knowledge budget" is now eaten up by inflated "indirect" or institutional overhead costs. You think you are buying a billion dollars worth of new knowledge and you are really buying only $600 million. Dr. Maria New, the Institute tells you, has been refunded—her grant is now $52,000. But $20,000 of that grant goes to the institution where she does her work as indirect costs for such non-research items as heat or light or janitorial service.

And what about those younger people who are not quite as well established? A contract study for NIH is now investigating what has happened to 200 applicants whose grant proposals were approved but not funded. Although there are as yet no results, the impressions gained through preliminary interviews with 20 investigators tend to confirm the experiences of Doctors New, Deykin, Insull, Weil, Coulson and Levine. If researchers are established, they usually piece together support of some sort, and go on, although perhaps not in the exact same way they hoped to go. If they are comparatively young and not yet strengthened by long curriculum vitae and bibliographies, they may be on the way to being lost to research work and the potential results of a productive research career may be lost to society.

To see what other forces are shaping the researchers of the future, one must examine — or try to examine — the training of the researchers of today.

7.   The Future: Instability

If you were looking for someone to cast in the role of dedicated young medical researcher of today, you might pick Robert Wondergem—25 years old, tall, bearded, serious, and caught in the whirlpool of the government's research training policies. When he started his graduate work in physiology three years ago at the Medical College of Wisconsin (formerly the Marquette University School of Medicine), Wondergem paid his own way. Then, as was the custom with students of promise, his department picked up his support under its National Heart and Lung Institute cardiovascular research training grant. He got a $2400 a year, tax free stipend when he started his pre-doctoral work, hardly a munificent sum, but enough for a young investigator.

A year and a half into the program, Rob Wondergem and his fellow students heard perplexing news: the federal government was changing its training support policies; the training grant his Department of Physiology had held for fifteen years would not be renewed. The nature and demands of Rob's pre-doctoral work were such that he felt he could not both take a part time job and pursue his studies: he starts his laboratory work on hormonal problems at 7:30 or 8 in the morning and stays until 5 or 6 p.m.; following an intriguing lead he may stay until 9 p.m. several nights a week. Yet he and his young wife could not live on her small salary as a teacher in a private school.

113

Before the President's Biomedical Research Panel in Washington on the last day of June, in 1975, Paul O'Neill, Deputy Director of the White House's Office of Management and Budget, testified he found it very hard to assess the effect of the change in the government's research manpower training program. O'Neill held it was not yet abundantly clear whether or not the affected universities had diverted funds to keep the training program going, and thus meet the acid test as to the importance of various programmatic activities. In non-federal jargon, if the training were really necessary, the universities would take funds away from some other activity to support it.

It's a long way from such impersonal pronouncements in the throne room to those affected by them. Scrounging for support, a Wisconsin Heart Association fellowship here, a moonlighting job there, the Wisconsin program, led by Doctors James J. Smith, M.D. and Howard M. Klitgaard, Ph.D., did manage to salvage the thirty graduate students on their rolls the year the axe fell. In Rob's case, they talked a local Veterans' Administration team into hiring him as a technician. Had he been a humanities graduate student engaged largely in course work, a side job might have worked out. But as a scientist he felt uncomfortable killing a third of his time when his real work waited in the laboratory at school. He felt lucky when he later received one of two stipends his Department of Physiology was able to get through the Graduate Studies Council; now he will be able to complete his Ph.D. and start on a research career.

Still, such funds come nowhere near covering the costs (around $100,000 a year) of a program supporting not only pre- and post-doctoral trainees, but visiting faculty scholars and some summer and free time medical, dental and college level students. (The program trained 84 "pre-docs" and 46 "post-docs", 21 of them Ph.D.s, and 17 M.D.s, and 125 medical, dental or undergraduate non-degree scientists.) Pessimism prevails as to the future of a program whose chief interest is hormonal regulation of growth and development, and especially the effect of exercise on the heart. "Without

114

financial aid I am not interested", a prospective student writes.
Another reports, "I have been unsuccessful in raising sufficient
funds and for this reason I will be unable to attend your
university." A school without a sumptuous endowment may
find it difficult if not impossible to meet Paul O'Neill's acid test
and plan a graduate program. When a bright eyed, involved
student with a good research idea knocked at the Physiology
Department door recently and said she would like to work
there, faculty members invited her to join them but had to tell
her they did not have funds for her support. Inquiring into the
possibility of a fellowship from the NHLI under the National
Research Service Award Act of 1974, she found it would be
some months before a competition would be held and then
completed, and even after those months had passed, it would
not yet be clear whether the program had been renewed or
funded.

Try to figure this one out: the National Heart and Lung
Institute is now struggling to administer four separate,
overlapping training programs to train young investigators—
three on the way out, and a new one that got off the ground
briefly, and then faltered.

Telescoped, the training program mess, as many call it,
evolved this way. In January 1973, the Nixon Administration
decided to phase out the two traditional federal research
training programs for both pre-and post-doctoral students,
and impounded the funds that Congress had already
appropriated for their support. The two programs were:

The training grant, awarded to institutions which in turn
select and train health researchers; this program absorbed
most of the NIH research training funds;

The research fellowship, an award made directly to trainees
selected at NIH in national competition.

The NIHers reacted sharply; they perceived the phase-out
and impoundment as a hostile act. The bioscientific brouhaha
raised around the country was heard, both in the predominant-

ly Democratic Congress and to a lesser extent in the Republican Administration. As the health leaders on Capitol Hill held hearings, struggling to continue the programs, HEW started the "Weinberger" Program, named after the boss, HEW Secretary Caspar Weinberger, and emphasizing post-doctoral research training fellowships and awards in fields of critical need.

Next, a number of organizations representing professional schools, including the Association of American Medical Colleges, the American Association of Dental Schools and the American Association of Colleges of Pharmacy rallied around the flag. They brought separate suits in the federal courts for the restoration of impounded funds. The AAMC succeeded first and as a result of a final court decision in January, 1974, NIH got back the funds and was able to pick up almost where it had left off.

In this case, as in others where NIH had suffered at the hands of the Administration, the Congress came to the rescue. It restored the research training programs—with, as we shall see, some new twists of its own.

But National Heart and Lung Institute applicants did not escape from the labyrinth with the enactment of the new law. First it was delayed in a bureaucratic bottleneck: it took six months until regulations could be worked out and published in the Federal Register. No sooner could one competition be held, and the first set of 138 awards be made, than the one year authorization for the Act expired. A second set of applications passed through the dual peer review process. But these applicants—a group of 55 research fellows—did not get their training funds though the program was operating under a continuing resolution, because the NIH, under unwritten orders from OMB not to make new research grant and contract starts, had placed a moratorium on all such starts, and NHLI officials had interpreted this to include training awards.

Anticipating renewal of the new National Research Service Award Act, a third competition announced in October

1975 solicited applications with an early January 1976 deadline. But the announcement enclosed in kits mailed to prospective applicants bore this formidable caveat:

> The provisions of this announcement are subject to any changes which may be necessary as a result of Congressional action on pending legislation extending basic authorization for the program. Such awards will be contingent upon availability of funds.

Congress departed for its year-end holiday without completing action on the NIH research training measure, but not before President Ford had vetoed a long delayed Labor-HEW appropriations bill for the current year.

No wonder that confusion reigned, that university people found it hard to get coherent answers as to what funds might be available, and that young investigators puzzled as to whether they should bother to apply at all. The telephone calls to a Washington lobbyist for the medical schools persisted: "What's cooking on training grants?" He answered: "Call us next week." But next week he had to say he still didn't know.

NHLI Advisory Council member Dr. Eugene Braunwald, has labeled the debacle of the research training programs "scientific infanticide" and their sporadic funding "capricious". Around Washington it is known as the instability issue.

Some say this instability is a technical problem, and indeed it has its baffling mechanical aspects. The federal budget process is a complicated one; eighteen months lapse between the first drafting of budget requests and the beginning of a fiscal year. The span of the fiscal year will change in calendar 1976—instead of beginning July 1 it will begin on October 1 and the months between July and October 1976 are called the transition quarter or wedge period; fiscal year 1977 will begin on October 1, 1976; training programs are forward funded as much as a year in advance. (This year's funds are to support next year's trainees).

Congress must act twice in order to establish and fund a new program or to extend certain older ones. It must first pass an authorization act, which goes through committees having substantive jurisdiction over the subject matter. This law merely says that there shall be such and such a program and Congress may appropriate money for it. Then Congress must pass an appropriations act. In each house this is considered in detail by an appropriations subcommittee and approved by a full committee. The appropriations act does not usually appropriate as much money as was authorized. Programs may continue to operate without either authorization or appropriations or both, under a continuing resolution: a stopgap which provides money at the previous year's rate, or at the rate of the budget proposed by the President ("the President's level"), whichever is less, or at a still different rate.

The enactment of the Congressional Budget and Impoundment Control Act of 1974 was an effort to make the budget process more orderly. But it has unexpectedly raised new instabilities. A President may no longer on his own impound funds the Congress has authorized and appropriated. He may, however, defer, or ask Congress to rescind, the use of these funds: deferrals do not take effect if disapproved by either house, and rescissions have to be approved by both houses of Congress within 45 days or they do not take effect. Not many rescissions have actually been approved. But since it is difficult for Congress to act in 45 days, and no appropriated funds are spent within those 45 days, both rescissions and deferrals are at least temporarily effective budget paring tools, and President Ford has made use of them repeatedly in the health field.* At the close of 1975, the NIH Director's office sent out a budget guideline memorandum. Because of "the unknown

---

*Forty-three percent of the rescissions proposed in fiscal 1975 were for health programs, according to The Coalition for Health Funding, a five year old coordinating group of academic, professional and other groups that lobby for health appropriations.

problematic impact of potential deferrals and rescissions", there would continue to be no new research grants or contracts funded in the third quarter of that fiscal year.

But the instability issue transcends such technicalities. It is, in fact, a political issue. The biomedical community has been whipsawed between the Republican Administration and the Democratic Congress as one has tried to cut, the other to expand, redirect, or at least to continue social programming. A dialogue from the President's Biomedical Panel proceedings on June 30, 1975 underlines this point.

The two top Congressional staff men who deal with health appropriations testified before the group, chaired by Dr. Franklin Murphy (head of the Los Angeles Times-Mirror Corporation and former Chancellor of the University of Kansas and UCLA):

Mr. Neil (Henry Neil, staff, House Appropriations Subcommittee, Labor-HEW): Well, I believe that the basic reason for the instability that people are concerned about in the field of medical research is very simple. It is a difference of opinion between the legislative and the executive branch. And I don't think that it's a mechanical problem, that it is due to something wrong with procedures. I think it's just a difference of opinion . . .

Mr. Dirks (Harley Dirks, staff, Senate Appropriations Subcommittee, Labor-HEW): I agree with Henry, it is a matter of confrontation between the executive and legislative branches. It is a problem of selecting priorities. And there, again, it is not the mechanism but deciding the priorities of the nation. Is health a priority? And if the answer is yes in both branches, then I think we have a sound basis to proceed on it. But if we have to go through an annual turn-around on the veto process, the impoundment process, the rescission and deferral process, I think the biomedical community is the constant loser . . .

Chairman Murphy: The problem is 200 million Americans usually make that decision, either wisely or unwisely.

If the answer is yes in both branches. The date: March 20, 1973, two months after the Nixon impoundment. The place, Room 2212, Rayburn House Office Building.

The primary protagonist for the Administration's decision to upset the traditional training program was, all agreed, the OMB's Health Branch chief, Victor Zafra. Yet such is the impenetrability of the bureaucracy, that the witness testifying before the Subcommittee on Public Health and Environment was not Zafra, and not his chief at the OMB and not the Department of Health, Education, and Welfare's Secretary or Undersecretary or the Assistant Secretary for Health, but one Dr. John S. Zapp, a Deputy Assistant Secretary for Legislation in HEW. Upon the shoulders of this Republican dentist from Oregon who had earned his political spurs as a hard working fund raiser for the Nixon-Agnew campaign, was placed the burden of Mr. Nixon's decision—to be found illegal in court—to discontinue a program established for over two decades. He was accompanied by two equally uncomfortable veteran NIH men who were soon to leave their posts, Deputy Director John Sherman and Associate Director for Program Planning and Evaluation Dr. Thomas J. Kennedy.

Chairman Paul G. Rogers, a vigorous interrogator, spread on the record his concern about the absence of higher HEW officials and their apparent lack of interest in a major cog in the national health machine. He proceeded to show that Dr. Zapp had hardly been involved in the decision to end the research training program made sometime in November or December of 1972, and then subjected him to a barrage of questions.

Were there any surveys, any studies made? Was this—and Mr. Rogers held up the large turquoise Volume I of "The Training Programs of the National Institutes of Health Fiscal Year 1974"—part of the three year background study which the witness said had played a very significant part in justifying the end of the program?

The volume the Chairman displayed had never seen the

light of day until the Association of American Medical Colleges' Dr. Michael Ball (who was lobbying in support of research training) had surreptitiously obtained a supply of copies for committee members from the NIH training staff and piled them in the back of his car. It was one of many statistics-studded studies which attested to the usefulness of the programs: A blue ribbon, but never officially published* President's Science Advisory Committee (PSAC) report; several National Academy of Sciences reports prepared under contract for the NIGMS (National Institute of General Medical Sciences, the Institute which supported most of NIH's pre-doctoral training), thick, two-part analyses issued first in 1970, and again in 1972. All supported the research training and fellowship programs. All warned of the dangers of cutting off the program without what the PSAC report called the "creation of alternate mechanisms assuring an uninterrupted flow of research and teaching manpower for both basic and clinical science".

All of these reports had fallen on deaf ears, as Mr. Rogers proceeded to point out. He read off recommendations of the volume in his hand:

That direct support of the training of candidate biomedical scientists for careers in research be reaffirmed as an appropriate and necessary role for the federal government.

That the existing instrument of support, the graduate training grants and our research fellowships continue to be the key element in the NIH training programs.

That alternative proposals for producing the manpower required for the existing and contemplated levels of federally supported biomedical research seem upon analysis to be of dubious merit and potentially disastrous.

How the OMB had interpreted such recommendations

*The committee printed its conclusions and recommendations as an Appendix in House Report No. 93-224 on HR 7724, May 23, 1973.

Chairman Rogers did not know, nor did he appreciate the Administration alternatives—small basic educational grants for undergraduates and general support for research, some of which would go to apprentice bioscientists in a "free marketplace". Questioned by North Carolina's Representative Richardson Preyer, a former federal judge, Dr. Zapp set forth three Administration reasons for ending the training program. First, he thought, but was not sure, that a third of those trained had not continued careers in academic research—but he admitted a one third fallout was not unusual and the experience would have enhanced their medical skills in any case. Second, there were some indications of an excess of scientific manpower in some fields; more qualified people were submitting more qualified research applications and in three of 16 fields identified by NIGMS training committees (biophysics, biochemistry and physiology) the job market was approaching or had reached saturation. Third, sufficient numbers of bioscientists would enter research anyway without federal subsidy.

The Committee agreed with Congressman Preyer that Zapp's evidence was not based on hard data, and that the Administration had not carried the burden of proof. Weighing the arguments, its members and later their colleagues in the full House and Senate leaned toward—though they did not accept completely—all the views of all the NIHers. These views were hardly as unanimous as their cries of deep dismay.

Deans and academicians worried about the institutional training grants on which so many of their departments had been built and had come to depend. Many basic scientists were concerned about the fate of the individual fellowships supporting researchers. After all, in a sense, the training grant is an elitist mechanism, not every department in every one of the nation's 114 medical schools can have one. You need a mechanism to support promising young individual bioscientists on their own. What's more, physician-trainers feared for the future of clinical research: Society needs the skills of those doctors who study whole patients outside the laboratory—who else can use the high technology of modern medicine to plumb the human heart? Yet if that same society fails to support their research training it runs the risk of losing them to greener pastures. And who then, will do clinical research?

The Association of American Medical Colleges led the biomedical community's attempts to remedy the Administration decision, and worked with the Rogers staff to develop alternative legislation and line up hearing witnesses. Dr. Michael Ball, then director of that organization's Division of Biomedical Research, recalls the difficulty of coordinating diffuse groups of bioscientists whose approach to research training varied according to their vantage points. "It was a cacophony of sound", he remembers. Harvard spoke for Harvard, Old Boondocks for Old Boondocks.

Other observers, anonymous, of course, perceived in all these outcries a self-serving interest in protecting academic turf. One high NIH bureaucrat involved felt that too many people had lost sight of the overall common public good; "they had the gimmes". In his view, as in that of many others, the Office of Management and Budget could have gotten farther if it had gone about its effort to reduce the research training programs in a less high-handed, "Nixonian" way.

Essentially, the difference of opinion over the NIH research training programs centered on three questions: Is there a proper Federal role in the training of biomedical scientists? If there is such a role, how should the government determine what sort of scientists are needed in what areas? And through what mechanism should such support be funneled?

At the beginning, it seemed as though the Nixon Administration had decided to answer *no* to the first question and end research training programs as it had done in a similar government agency, the National Science Foundation. The phase-out of the research training programs and impoundment of their funds was developed largely at the White House's

Office of Management and Budget and sold against the advice of his science advisers to a President eager to reduce government spending and not particularly enamoured of academia, medical or otherwise. Testifying before the Biomedical Research Panel session on June 30, 1975, OMB Deputy Director Paul O'Neill explained that "looking at what we are doing across the government in support of training of all kinds, the President decided that what we were doing was inequitable and in a lot of different ways, and yes, decided we weren't going to do this any more." He added that biomedical research training was the last remaining area where the federal government is providing funds for the ostensible purpose of training research people.

Behind such words as "inequitable" and "ostensible" lie several arguments which grew familiar in the early 1970s as the NIHers strove to respond to a series of OMB questions about the programs: What were their objectives? How many of each type of trainee were being supported? How could shortages be measured and could such shortages or oversupply be identified in any specialty?

The public policy or equity argument held that the federal government does not support training in such other fields as law or accounting, why should it do so in bioscience—a fat field akin to medicine and enjoying many of the benefits Americans offer in return for better health care. The Nixon Administration was paring funds going to all of academia, and trying to substitute repayable loans and limit grants to the needy. Why should research be exempt? What's more, the programs were admittedly supplying training for at least some young physicians who ultimately would spend less time in research than in highly paid private practice. This was more true in some fields—like psychiatry or cardiovascular physiology—where the need for personnel had at one point seemed extreme. Why should a $12,000 a year bus driver-taxpayer contribute to the training of professionals who would be earning very high incomes throughout their careers? Or why should he contribute to the support of research fellows who did some research but spent a great deal of training time taking care of patients—in many cases, as one physician who worked with them observed, private patients of big men who have a great easy life and get rich too?

Another argument contended that the federal training programs had supplied the nation with sufficient biomedical scientists; the market for their services was limited; it is poor policy to train people for jobs which may not materialize. Enough engineers were driving taxicabs as it was as a result of post-Sputnik enthusiasm for engineering; it would be foolish to support more biochemists only to have them join the ranks. Better, let demand and supply work their will in the marketplace, leading the right number of people to get themselves trained in the right fields. There is a deeper dimension to this argument: Back to that June 30, 1975 Biomedical Research panel meeting and the questioning of the OMB Deputy Director:

Dr. Ebert (Dean Robert H. Ebert of Harvard Medical School): In other words, is it (the decision which gets made with regard to research manpower) based on a projection that if you train more manpower there will be more funds needed for more programs and the whole thing will continue to escalate? . . . Is there a feeling that this area of training no longer needs subsidy because it will propel itself?

Mr. O'Neill: Well, it is a complex of things that you have suggested and it is also, I think, fair to say, that kind of decision is driven by fiscal pressure.

The market for research had stabilized, the argument ran, pressure on the health dollar was increasing; it was needed for other health services. Once you train bioscientists you will probably have to support them throughout their careers through other federally funded programs. It would be wiser to turn off the funding-fountain before it was too late.

Answering, the NIH supporters pointed out that the American public has repeatedly demonstrated its desire for better health care and its willingness to pay for new discoveries.

Better health care implies a steady flow of medical research findings, of vaccines that prevent and drugs and surgical techniques that will cure. A vigorous biomedical research program is a matter of urgent national concern. In other fields of national concern, as in the military, where the federal government accepts a central role in funding, it also accepts responsibility for training. It has accepted a central role in the funding of medical research, as it has not done in law or accounting, so it should accept responsibility for training.

New researchers must be continuously trained, the NIHers argued. Research and training, trainer and student are inextricably bound together: how can you separate training for pure research from training for other less altruistic and more lucrative academic and medical practice activities for which the OMB considered federal support inappropriate? New investigators must be trained not only to fill the shoes of older men and women but because in their apprenticeship years they perform much of the hard work. Not everyone is cut out for a research career—it is during these years they find out if they have the necessary disciplined imagination, patience and persistence. Later, as they begin to become established on their own, they usually must find a teaching base. Here they cannot succeed unless they publish and cannot publish unless they do research.

The training pipeline is long—five or six years, on the average, for a Ph.D., ten years or more for the M.D. researcher and not everyone survives. You cannot turn the pipeline on and off—the flow must have a steady pressure. Research is a young person's game. A scientist usually reaches the age of 35 or so before he has sharpened his research tools, and become established as an independent investigator, on his own research path. Even then, he is apt to have a productive scientific lifetime of only about ten to a dozen years; it is the unusual person who is still in the laboratory at 65; by the time most reach 45 they may be so well known that they are distracted by service on innumerable committees. Or they may simply run

126

out of creative research ideas and turn to administrative or teaching work.

As Dr. Ephraim Friedman, then Dean of the Boston University School of Medicine, put it, the training programs in question may be looked on as medicine's seed crop, our investment in the future: "To consume a seed crop or slaughter breeding stock in time of famine is deplorable, but understandable. To do so at any other time is shortsighted, irrational, and in the case of this society at this time, simply obscene." The rate of return to a medical researcher on a training investment is low enough—especially, comparatively speaking, in the case of physicians—that society must invest in the support not of all, but of a reasonable number of bioscientists. Society must invest in the maintenance of first rate training institutions, to assure the continued vitality of the biomedical research program. This is too important a matter to leave to the uncertainties of the market place or the magnetism of current fads.

Admittedly, the job of pinpointing exactly how much of what kind of skills would be needed in ten or twenty years is extraordinarily difficult, when you do not know the extent of the country's research effort, or what new needs new discoveries will create. But the most fairminded among the NIHers accepted the notion that such an attempt could and should be made. It would be a human tragedy to train a bioscientist for long years only to find him unable to use his skills productively.

By the end of June, when Senate Subcommittee on Health Chairman Edward Kennedy opened hearings on a research training measure, the Administration had changed its tune. Dr. John S. Zapp was back on the Hill again, but this time with the Assistant Secretary for Health, Dr. Charles C. Edwards, who respectfully asked to modify the Administration's position. The time had come for a lateral pass. A few weeks later, Deputy Assistant Secretary for Health Henry E. Simmons testified

127

that though the Administration still opposed the Congressional measure, HEW Secretary Weinberger had announced a new program emphasizing post-doctoral fellows and training for areas of national need. (The "Weinberger fellowships".)

Another part of the picture which should be noted here was the role of Capitol Hill staff—a prominent ingredient in Washington conversation but one that is seldom publicly acknowledged.* This role has grown in recent years as Congress has sought to strengthen its impact on the $118 billion health care system, and to combat just such an antagonistic Nixon health policy as the research training phase-out and impoundment.

It used to be that Senators and Congressmen would simply call an official like HEW Secretary Wilbur Cohen for technical advice and politically marketable ideas. (Cohen had been HEW Undersecretary and before that, Assistant Secretary for Legislation and long before that had worked his way up the ladder of the Social Security Administration.) Now Congress had to build its own batteries of expertise. Writing in "National Journal Reports" in 1975,** John K. Iglehart reported that only six years ago the number of professional staff members on the four House and Senate authorizing committees and two appropriations subcommittees that write virtually all federal health legislation could be counted on one

---

*But is frequently described in scholarly publications. In "The Department of HEW", (Praeger Publishers 1974), Rufus Miles contends that the Clinical Center surgical wing completed in 1963 should have ben named the "Herman Downey Surgical Theater" after Senator Lister Hill's appropriations subcommittee clerk, a "gruff Tennessean who probably put more of his own initiative and talent for kibitzing into the construction than into any other aspect of NIH".

**See also the thorough description of Congressional health staff by John K. Iglehart, in "National Journal Reports", May 17, 1975.

hand: now their number is 26 and still growing. Several ancillary agencies—the Congressional Research Service and the General Accounting Office—have strengthened their health staffs. Moreover, the Congress has set up its own Office of Technology Assessment and Budget Offices and asked the National Academy of Sciences to conduct several in-depth health studies. And the Robert Wood Johnson Foundation enables a small group of select medical school faculty to work side by side with other health staff on Capitol Hill.

Quite naturally, many members of the new Congressional stable come from the Department of Health, Education, and Welfare to work on the other, more activist side of the fence. The Congressional ambience is attractive for many reasons. It is certainly less anonymous and impersonal, and often more fun than the huge faceless executive branch. Hill staffers usually enjoy their role at the elbow of power. On the Senate side especially, where members are fewer and spread thinner over a variety of issues, some of that power rubs off on them as their bosses depend on their knowledge and hard work. But they all work for successful politicians, and they learn early that credit is the name of the game. The boss gets it, and you work in tandem or he will not be your boss much longer.

Such nuances are not always well understood by medical newcomers to the growing health political arena whose political education may have stopped with high school civics. They are apt to suspect Byzantine intrigue especially among some of the young doctors on the Senate Health Subcommittee staff they consider inexperienced and overly assertive. At an early Biomedical Research Panel session in 1975, two former Nixon Assistant Secretaries for Health testified to the power of such staff "young people". Drawing a spidery array of lines and boxes on a flip pad with a magic marker, silver-haired Dr. Merlin K. DuVal, for one, led his audience through a paranoid nightmare, wherein staff worked first in HEW, then perhaps, for various health lobbies, then for legislative offices, leapfrogging over their bosses in a sort of conspiracy to effectuate plans for social engineering.

129

Most found this unrealistic: Senators and Congressmen are rarely puppets on any staff man's knee. In any case, the lobbyists for the NIHers, seeking a reinstatement of the NIH research training programs and led by the Association of American Medical Colleges found smoother sailing working with the Rogers than the Kennedy subcommittee staffs, represented, respectively, by Stephan Lawton and Dr. Lawrence Horowitz. Substance was involved: more in the traditional mould, the Rogers group included both full blown institutional training grants for medical school departments and individual fellowships in its proposed program, as the AAMC naturally preferred, and Kennedy's Committee emphasized the individual fellowships.

But it was more a question of style: Michael Ball remembers Larry Horowitz calling him and AAMC President Dr. John A.D. Cooper to Capitol Hill one day in June of 1973 and advising them curtly that either they took the ethics provision or they had no research training bill. Horowitz was referring here to Senator Kennedy's interest in protecting human research subjects who had been involved in questionable research projects of different kinds (the Senator's headlined hearings had spotlighted abuses like those in the HEW—but not NIH—supported long term Tuskegee syphilis study, where informed consent was lacking and patients were not treated with penicillin even after it became available.) Horowitz' version of the meeting differs: the AAMC men wanted a bill on an emergency basis because research training could not wait. He told them the Senator could not drop his high priority hearings on the ethics measure proposing a commission to study the protection of human research subjects, and he could not simply adopt a research training measure which in his judgment needed some revision without holding substantive hearings. The best way to get research training was to link it with the ethics measure.

The House leaders, for their part, wanted to call the Administration to heel on the research training measure swiftly. They feared if they mixed it with the ethics or human subjects issue, it might go down in the sticky controversial mire of abortion arguments, which were tied up with the problem of fetal research. But when the research training bill reached the House floor in late May of 1973, they did indeed find it necessary to bow to New York's Representative Angelo D. Roncallo, and include his amendment forbidding the Secretary of Health, Education, and Welfare to conduct research on a human fetus with a beating heart, outside the mother's uterus (what the experts call an abortus). As Interstate and Foreign Commerce Committee Chairman Harley Staggers put it: "Mr. Speaker, I am sorry this amendment passed. I voted for it because I did not want some demagogue to say I voted for experimentation on fetuses." He pointed out that the Committee bill already contained broad strictures against HEW research which violated ethical standards and that these strictures were in fact weakened by language which singled out one problem and ignored others, like those exemplified in the Tuskegee Study. The research training bill was approved by a vote of 361-5.

Summer passed; what Woodrow Wilson called "the dance of legislation" continued. The Senate health subcommittee interrupted its hearings on the protection of human subjects measure to hold two days of hearings on a new Kennedy research training measure. When the full Labor and Public Welfare Committee "marked up" the measures or cast them in concrete as one bill, it included the substance of Minnesota Senator Walter Mondale's S.J. Res. 71 directing the proposed commission for the protection of human subjects to undertake a comprehensive study of the ethical, social and legal implications of advances in biomedical and behavioral research and technology. On September 11, 1973, the National Research Service Award and Protection of Human Subjects Act passed the Senate by a vote of 81-6. On the floor, it was amended to include fetal research and psychosurgery as subjects for Commission study. New York Senator James L.

Buckley's amendment placing a ban on fetal research was compromised to become a temporary moratorium pending the recommendation of policies by the new commission four months after it was established.

With an eye to the House-Senate conference, Chairman Paul Rogers formulated his ideas on a commission for the protection of human subjects in still another bill and in late September, Senator Kennedy came over to the House side to testify as to its merits before the House Public Health and Environment subcommittee. The two leaders disagreed on certain aspects of this measure (as they had on aspects of research training itself): Kennedy wanted an independent, permanent body; Rogers a study group more accountable to HEW and the Congress.

Meanwhile, the challenge to the Nixon impoundment of the research training funds was moving through the courts. At length the Court of Appeals of the District of Columbia made it clear in January of 1974 that this impoundment was illegal and that the appropriated funds must be expended as provided by law. By February, NIH had put notices to this effect in the mail and the heat was off both houses to compromise their measures in conference to produce a new research training program quickly.

So it was not until July 12 that the National Research Service Award Act of 1974 became law. In the end, the Congress established a National Commission for the Protection of Human Subjects as Title II. This Commission was to be a two year body appointed by the Secretary of HEW; it was to be succeeded by a permanent National Advisory Council.

As for research training, Title I, the Congress wrote into the new law the finding that the success and continued viability of biomedical and behavioral research depends on the availability of excellent scientists and a network of institutions of excellence capable of producing superior research personnel. And it found that direct support of the training of scientists for research careers is an appropriate and necessary role for the Federal government.

But in hammering out the new measure, in making it acceptable to those who thought it reasonable and proper to tighten the programs and those who thought it necessary to do so to keep the Administration from emasculating them, the Congress changed their thrust and made them much less flexible. It compromised the House Rogers and the Senate Kennedy versions with these results:

First, the new $207 million program embodied more of the Administration's individualistic, no-free-lunch philosophy. It emphasized the individual trainee and his or her obligation to repay the society which supported his training. Under the old programs, the National Heart and Lung Institute had; like its sister institutes, put a significant portion of its training funds into improving the academic environment where training took place and setting national standards for it through long term, centrally reviewed and awarded institutional grants. This meant small stipends for students and general support for staff, equipment, and other such costs.

Now, there was to be more attention paid to the individual student, and a firmer hand on the federal spigot. At least 25 percent of the funds had to go for individual fellowships. A three year limit on the support of any one researcher aimed to funnel funds to researchers already one year into their work and thus committed to it (subject, however, to a waiver). A mandate that the HEW Secretary, through the National Academy of Sciences, undertake a broad continuing study to determine where medical researchers are needed, seeks eventually to confine training to those fields in which there is a need for personnel. (Thus far, the NAS has told NIH to continue the sort of training it is doing pending further in-depth studies.)

What's more, Congress attached short strings to the training awards. Recipients have to repay society for each

133

month of training by a month of research or teaching or public service in such places as the city slums, remote rural communities, or health maintenance organizations. Those who do not repay in service have to repay in money with accrued interest, according to a bewilderingly complex formula, and may end up paying substantially more than they receive. A young physician applying for a fellowship under the new pay-back formula has many paths open to him if his research career does not work out; non-physician scientists may be discouraged from applying, fearing they may end up teaching high school science for a modest salary, heavily in debt.

In one other important new way, the research training programs were sharply refocused on research. Research training has always been just that—research training. But most of the training programs supported by an Institute like NHLI, dealing with the critical human problems of heart disease, involve some clinical or people-centered activities. Seeking to avoid research training which might support young physicians who put substantial time into patient treatment and also provide them with lucrative specialized skills for the future, the new act specifically denied support to residencies. This meant no support for new doctors seeking further training (the internship—a year's hospital training before hanging out a shingle—has virtually disappeared in the last few years and become a part of a longer, more sophisticated medical center residency lasting at least three years).

But in the final days of work on the measure, NIH technicians had pointed out that in trying to plug the clinical leak, the Congress had taken away from NIH all authority to train clinicians, and should research produce new discoveries the agency would be left without a way to train doctors to apply them quickly to human ills. Although the legislators did restore the word "clinical" to the training program authorizations, NHLI peer reviewers have interpreted the new act's research intent strictly. Clinical programs unable or unwilling to tailor

134

their contents to pure research accordingly have lost out.

Dr. Proctor Harvey, a white haired gentleman with a pronounced southern accent, runs one of these. He has trained "post-docs" or new physicians who are interested in acquiring research tools in the field of cardiology at Georgetown Medical Center in Washington, D.C. for the past 26 years. His clinical program has enjoyed an excellent reputation, competition to enter has been stiff and it has trained about 120 "superb doctors", almost three-quarters of whom have gone into university based academic medicine, in this country and abroad. Like pebbles dropped into water, each of them has influenced others to teach and do research. Would not most patients seriously sick with heart disease prefer their services and would not future patients profit from their investigations?

Dr. Harvey does not know who made the decision that changed the government's training policies, Congress or the Administration, but he feels the change set medicine back 20 years. Another clinical investigator who lost his NHLI training grant, Dr. Benjamin Burrows of the University of Arizona College of Medicine, points to a paradox in new research training policies: though national leaders say they want new cures which can be applied to people, they have effectively limited support to those pursuing research and thus inhibited the very young physicians who in the future must shoulder most of the responsibility for applied research. And in his respiratory sciences field, there is even now a shortage of researchers and clinicians.

One hears worries from many different sources. Like many basic scientists, Dr. Ronald W. Estabrook, Dean of the Graduate School of Biomedical Sciences at the University of Texas Health Science Center in Dallas, is most concerned about training a steady flow of excellent, enthusiastic, knowledgeable research fellows to "fill in the necessary cracks between the bricks of the institutional programs". A biochemist, Dr. Estabrook explains that a department of radiology seeking new ways to examine a patient who had suffered a heart attack, for instance, would need a trained biochemist to find a substance with which to stain and then scan heart tissues. Today, it takes a very determined, dedicated individual to decide on such a research career.

Dr. Estabrook approves the new thrust: preparing for fields like epidemiology or biostatistics where there is a need for new investigators and fostering interdisciplinary training. But another basic scientist, Dr. Arthur C. Guyton, a former NHLI Council member and the current President of the 14,000-member Federation of American Societies for Experimental Biology feels that the new law, allowing individuals to be trained only for certain fields where they are needed, has had a restrictive effect. The old program used to allow young investigators to train where they felt good work was being done. Now he reports, on visits to medical centers throughout the country he has seen an amazing number of people working not where their interest is, but where the federal dollar lies. Herding trainees into targeted areas for which they are not motivated, he warns, can dim the spark of genius.

Dr. Guyton, a well known physiologist who is Chairman of the University of Mississippi Medical Center's Department of Physiology and Biophysics, is concerned about the increasing inability of medical school departments in less developed parts of the country to compete for training funds— as budgets squeeze, the rich and well-established who have historically attracted the topmost talent get richer and more established. Hearing this, a community-minded physician answers, "Great! Maybe those who don't get research grants will train clinicians to work out in the country where they are needed. Do they want everyone in medicine to be a researcher?" And he adds that many leaders of the bioscientific community argue against the market mechanism, but still find it hard to accept intelligent planning.

In the last analysis, the research training problem in the mid-1970s is not so much the changes in program format, nor the lessening of federal funding, but the unstable nature of the federal funding that now exists.

Before the big change, the National Heart and Lung Institute was supporting 1,389 full time trainees in all its research training programs, at a cost of $19.6 million. Afterwards, in 1975, the expanded Institute was supporting 1,173 at a cost of $19.3 million (both an inflation-generated increase in training stipends and the abrupt restoration of impounded funds contributed to this total). But 618 of these 1,173 trainees—either in the old institutional (552) or fellowship (10) or Weinberger fellowship (56) programs will have been phased out within the next three years.

New trainees could take their place, under the National Research Service Award Act, but many were skeptical of the powers of that on-again, off-again law, in a time of budgetary austerity. At Peter Bent Brigham Hospital in Boston, Dr. Eugene Braunwald reports he spends as much as an hour a day counseling students. He is involved in career decisions; students interested in research come to him, discouraged, not about the amounts of money, but about the uncertainty of a future in teaching and research. Dr. Braunwald headed a notable group* of research training advocates who now accept the need for a formalized mechanism for the study of scientific manpower which could analyze the flow of scientific personnel on the one hand and shortages in specific disciplines, on the other, and then make periodic decisons about launching new programs and curtailing others. Although he advises his students to hang in there until the dust settles, he cannot blame promising young people who have many, many options— including the lucrative private practice of cardiology—when

*See Dr. Braunwald's "The Training of Manpower Needed for Biomedical Research", in the *New England Journal of Medicine*, Feb. 6, 1975. This article was submitted on behalf of the American Society for Clinical Investigation's Committee on National Medical Policy.

they turn away from a commitment to research. "Understandably", he told a House of Representatives health subcommittee, they are "unwilling to throw their lot in with a system which gyrates as wildly as the biomedical research enterprise."

If there were a steady flow of funds through NIH—no matter the size or formulation—the trainers would accommodate themselves to such changes, local program directors who did get institutional grants would be able to admit a definite number of students each year, young investigators would be able to figure out when to apply for what, and how. All of them might complain at times, but if the flow were steady they could plan ahead and work efficiently.

But there is no such steady flow. One day there are funds, the next day there are none. One day a research training program is there, the next day it is not. Long discouraging lags between application and grant awards make it hard, if not impossible, to plan ahead. Congress says *yes* and has kept the training programs alive; the White House says *no*—it has preferred to let them die.

The losers may be the young investigators in the heartland of America who find it hard both to pursue a research career and stay afloat. Or they may be you and me—the patients waiting for a new vaccine, a new drug, a new approach to the prevention of heart disease or cancer. Such a discovery would, in all probability, come from a young researcher probing basic problems on the far borders of bioscience.

8.   The Totally Implantable Artificial Heart:

The "Impossible" Decisions

In your chest, toward the front and left, beats a remarkable pump: the human heart. Simple, yet sophisticated in design, enduring, hard working, efficient and quiet, yet usually attracting attention only in the event of dramatic failure, it squeezes and relaxes 70 to 80 times a minute, 100,000 times every 24 hours, 36 million times a year, pushing 16,000 quarts of blood through 60,000 miles of blood vessels each day.

This muscular, four chambered organ about the size of your fist is really two pumps in one, with four valves preventing blood from flowing in the wrong direction. Each side, or pump, does a different job. Without oxygen, your body cells would suffocate; the right side pumps oxygen-poor blood from the body into the lungs; the left side collects oxygen-enriched blood from the lungs and pumps it to the body. Using chemical energy released when the blood sugars and oxygen combine, the heart pays attention to all of life's vagaries, without any help from you. It speeds up automatically when you need energy to run to catch the bus, or to fight, out of fear or anger. It slows down when you rest, when you feel cool, contented or calm.

The heart surpasses modern technology's most advanced machines. Yet throughout history, men and women have regarded it in quite a different light—not as a pump, but as the seat of noble emotions, of courage, of joy, or of charity, and of course, of love. More than the brain, they have considered it central to rational and irrational life. Blaise Pascal, supreme logician, regarded it with reverence: "The heart has its reasons which reason knows nothing of." No wonder, then, that as medicine has leapt forward in this century, they have thought the idea of replacing a diseased or injured leg, or set of teeth, or breast, or even kidney, far less audacious than replacing the heart with a man-made prosthesis—an apparatus suitable for the Tin Woodman of Oz, or for a science fiction character, but not for you and me.

Yet, in the early fifties a new instrument, the heart-lung machine, permitted investigators in scattered laboratories to begin the search for such an artificial heart and their work led to a stepped up, coordinated effort under the National Heart Institute's leadership involving physicians, scientists, designers, technicians, and engineers at medical centers and industrial firms around the country. This search has not been long, in terms of even one lifetime on this planet. Nor has it been free of steep scientific hurdles. The innovators have had to design a pump, and an engine to drive that pump, and a power source for the engine. They have had to devise some sort of electronic control system to keep the heart delicately attuned to the pace of human life, and most difficult, to find biomaterials with which to line the pump—materials which would not injure blood, that most vulnerable fluid, and cause it to clot. They needed, too, to construct the heart out of a substance durable yet flexible enough to survive the heart's constant squeezing and relaxing motions. Then they had to fit all the parts together, develop the total configuration, and test it in animals to see if it would work therapeutically in living creatures.

There is no totally implantable artificial heart (TIAH) today. Only prototypes exist, usually four chambered pumps about the size of the natural heart, made of plastic and metals, powered by electrical, pneumatic or nuclear energy and electronically controlled; some are lined with flocked dacron velour, a soft velvety material. All the parts have been tested *successfully in animals, and by 1972, when the National Heart, Blood Vessel, Lung, and Blood Act was enacted, and the Institute's program broadened and expanded, it seemed as though the researchers had finished with feasibility studies and were about to enter the final pre-clinical phase. It seemed as though they might be on their way to perfecting such a heart for the estimated 16,750 to 50,300 desperately sick heart disease patients who might benefit from its implantation each year.*

Instead, official interest lagged: the program, which had been severely contained from the beginning, was, as the bureaucrats say, "deemphasized". Some say that this is only a detour on the admittedly long road to the solution of an intricate biological and engineering problem, a detour forced by budget stringencies. Others say it is more than that. They feel the artificial heart can be made to work inside the chests of human beings, if not in this decade, then in the next, and if this does not come to pass, it will be because the effort has not equalled the task. It will be because society has hung back, fearful of the tough social and ethical questions involved.

Who, for example, would pay the price for each heart— surely $15,000 to $25,000, plus maintenance? Would government be willing to cover its costs, as it has chosen to do for kidney transplants and dialysis? Who would participate in the great adventure of the clinical trials which must precede the heart's widespread use? Once the heart proved clinically acceptable, once mass-produced, would everyone among those critically ill with heart disease get one? If this is not possible, who would make this gift of life, and on what basis? With an artificial heart beating away inside, would the quality of a recipient's life actually be improved? Puzzling too, what is the interface between life and death? What is the meaning, the definition, of a death suffered when the heart continues to pound away inside the body? In view of all the complexities, is TIAH worth developing at all?

Such are the impossible decisions. Such are the social choices posed by the impingement of just such a technological

141

and scientific development as TIAH. Such are the social decisions that transcend scientific skill and now must confront us all.

We are back now, in the golden years of the sixties, when a Congress impatient for medical breakthroughs treated NIH with great generosity. We are back in that fabled era when NIH public information people would set up exhibits at scientific meetings to encourage grant applications. Dr. Ralph E. Knutti, now a 74-year-old retired medical administrator in a Maryland suburban rambler, reflects on those days when as director of the National Heart Institute: "Frankly, we had more money than we knew what to do with." One year, he remembers, his Institute had to return $17 million to the federal treasury which it had received too late to spend intelligently.

On February 18, 1965, House Health Appropriations Subcommittee Chairman John Fogarty was questioning Dr. Knutti about the budget proposed for the next fiscal year, in his detailed, nitty gritty way. "It is not much of a budget," Mr. Fogarty observed. He reminded the witness that last year in its report, the Committee expressed the opinion that more effort should be put into the artificial heart. What had the Institute done about it?

"We have not been sitting still in this respect," Dr. Knutti advised the Chairman. Institute funding over a number of years, he pointed out, had supported grantees developing heart-lung machines, surgical techniques to correct congenital heart disease, and a better understanding of cardiac and circulatory physiology. All this, he explained, had contributed to the present situation in which an advisory group composed of some of the country's leading cardiovascular investigators and practitioners had expressed its conviction that devices for partial or temporary assistance to the failing heart or even a total implantable replacement are desirable and feasible objectives to pursue. The advisory group had recommended that the Institute move with a sense of urgency since the devices could substantially benefit many patients afflicted by heart disease.

This did not satisfy Mr. Fogarty. How much money did the group recommend? How much would it cost? Did the Institute Director think it a feasible project to pursue, or to get started on?

The doctor thought it difficult to assign a specific price tag, though ultimately it would cost a tremendous amount of money. A caveat: the most important development problems now were engineering or technological, not purely physiological or surgical. Certain adjustments had to be made; the Heart Institute needed technical staff which could speak the same language as industrial and engineering experts. Contracts would have to be used, and the contract mechanism streamlined to make it more efficient. In other words, the Institute would have to enter into a mode of research and development similar to that used by the Air Force, the Atomic Energy Commission, or the National Aeronautics and Space Administration.

This still did not satisfy Mr. Fogarty. He had been told that there was solid basis for expecting the heart in 10 years. He had had a letter from Nobel laureate Dr. Joshua Lederberg at Stanford Medical School who just could not understand why we had not made more progress. Could it be done in 10 years, 5 years?

Dr. Knutti: If we go about this thing in order to develop a workable artifical assist to the circulation and want to get it done promptly and don't want to hold it back . . . five to ten years.

Mr. Fogarty: . . . Put it at this point in the record. I am convinced that something can be done in this field. I assume it is going to cost a lot of money, but I am getting tired of voting for bills for foreign aid, the farm programs, and getting a man on the moon, when we quibble over a few million dollars in trying to develop an artificial heart.

Spurred on by such Congressional appetite for discovery,

one would think that the Institute would have swung into high gear. One would think its Director would have received all the support he needed to launch, and sustain, a moon-shot or heart-shot effort. To see why this did not come to pass, it is necessary to look back at the four periods into which the story of the totally implantable artificial heart can be divided: First, the very early days: through 1965. Second, containment: the limited beginning of the NIH artificial heart program and its exploration of the separate pathways that might lead to a total heart (1966-1968). Third, cardiowizardry: the reaction to the wave of heart transplants which followed Dr. Christiaan Barnard's first operations in Cape Town, Dr. Denton Cooley's brief implantaton of an artificial heart in a patient; the effort to put together first the Left Ventricular Assist Device (LVAD) and then a total heart (TIAH) and test them in animals. Concern for the social and ethical questions involved. (1969-1972). Fourth, "The Ethics Report" and deemphasis: the highlighting of the impossible decisions and the deemphasis of the quest for TIAH. (1973-present).

The early days: The development, in mid-century, of the heart-lung machine, gave investigators and practitioners concerned with that most critical of national health problems, heart disease, the chance to dream and begin work on a variety of devices which might eventually help, or even replace, the human heart. This impressive machine takes over the heart's job, for a time at least, oxygenates blood outside the body, and allows the surgeon to open the chest and work in and around the heart in a quiet and "dry" or blood-free field.

In scattered laboratories, scientists conducted many different animal experiments—here they worked on an implanted, pneumatically driven blood pump, there on an external booster pump. Dr. Knutti remembers flying to Ohio during this period to meet with the developer of the artificial kidney machine, Dr. Willem J. Kolff, who, with his group at the Cleveland Clinic Foundation, had implanted an artificial heart first in dogs, and then more successfully but for very short periods, in calves. The doctor still has a picture of this event around the house. (The calf, whose circulatory system most closely resembles man's, became a more favored animal for these experiments than the dog, sheep, or mini-pig.)

The impetus to coordinate such separate efforts, give them technological and industrial backup, and transform them into a single high priority program came in the fall of 1963 from the National Heart Advisory Council and its planning committee. Pursuing the Council's interests—which in turn reflected those of the individual investigators involved—Dr. Knutti appointed the all-star advisory group he had quoted to Mr. Fogarty, which included Dr. Michael E. De Bakey and such other well-known names as Doctors Cowles E. Andrus, Eugene Braunwald, and Willem Kolff. This advisory group—a time honored way of both getting powerful scientific advice, and conferring outside approval on bureaucratic decision making—gave the artificial heart program its real go ahead and initial sense of urgency.

The space program was the exemplar in those days, the systems development approach the way to chart any strange ocean. Setting up the new artificial heart program office, Dr. Knutti looked for and found a physician with industrial experience and contacts, Dr. John R. Beem, medical research director for the Warner-Lambert pharmaceutical firm. The NHI men talked with many people dealing with specific systems development projects at the AEC, the DOD, and NASA. A dedicated Quaker physician and pioneer artificial heart researcher, Dr. Frank Hastings, joined up in the summer of 1964, and as the small staff developed it recruited still another advisory committee. This one included such R&D experts as the Air Force's General Bernard Schriever and NASA's Hugh Dryden. An Air Force Colonel was assigned to assist and Dr. DeBakey sent one of his young men up from Houston to help out.

Meanwhile, Dr. Beem had asked Institute grantees working in the field to suggest problems which could be attacked through the contract mechanism and whose solution would be useful to them. The NHI sought special permission to consider contracts and soon announced a number of contract opportunities through *Commerce Business Daily*. The nine resulting contracts, awarded in 1964, among the first non-drug contracts in NIH research, cost about a half million dollars, and covered such tasks as the development of pumps, drive units, mock circulating systems, and blood compatible materials. Seeking to lay a broad base for a systems approach to the artificial heart, the Institute, a year later, awarded another six contracts costing another half million dollars. With this funding, medical engineering teams based at the laboratories of various industrial giants like Westinghouse, or the Stanford Research Institute, and involving local community hospitals, worked to try to find out what technology did and did not exist in the field, what sort of resources and manpower might be needed, and what personal and social problems might be involved in the development of an artificial heart. Since NHI did not have the expertise to evaluate their massive findings, it contracted with a consulting firm, Hittman Associates of Baltimore, to do so.

Toward the close of his questioning of NHI Director Knutti in mid-February of 1965, Chairman Fogarty asked for a complete statement of how much money would be needed in addition to what was already in the budget to develop an artificial heart, and what structural changes would have to be made to allow the Institute to go ahead with such a program.

Dr. Beem and his associates complied. Their proposed master plan for artificial heart development was included in the record of that hearing. It laid out a four phase plan for producing the heart in five years' time. The total cost was estimated at about $40 million, including $300,000 for the rest of fiscal year 1965, $2.2 million in fiscal 1966, $17 million for fiscal 1967, and $20 million in fiscal 1968; (firmer and more precise predictions would be made as the plan proceeded). February 14, 1970, Valentine's Day, was to be Heart Sunday, the day the total artificial heart was certified for use.

They also asked for "no year" funding and Congressional recognition of the need to modify the traditional approach to NIH research. What they were really asking for was a miniature forerunner of the War on Cancer.

Containment: Instead NIH got, or quietly created, a program limited both in size and concept. Dr. Knutti had held out the hope of a program in five years, "if we don't want to hold it back."

The NIH chose to hold it back. Its leaders took the fiscal 1967 funds the Congress gave them for the artificial heart program—$13.7 million—and divided them: $8.7 million for the artificial heart, the rest for a new sister program to study myocardial infarction or heart attacks. (Some sarcastically referred to this division as "the rape of the artificial heart program".) The program became, not Mr. Fogarty's vision of the concentrated moonshot to develop an artificial heart, but a diversified effort aiming to create a family of devices to support the failing heart.

This remarkable transformation took place without fanfare and without, so far as can be determined, any Congressional criticism. 1966 was the decisive year—a confused period not only for the artificial heart program, now headed by Dr. Frank Hastings, but for the whole National Heart Institute. Dr. Knutti retired from his position as NHI director in July of 1965 and between that date and November of 1966 when Dr. Donald Fredrickson took over, the NHI had five different permanent and acting chiefs. The man who actually presided over the program split, Dr. Robert Grant, died after only six months in office.

But the decision to contain the artificial heart program is known to this day as "Dr. Shannon's decision". It was NIH director Dr. James Shannon who sent word from Building One that NHI should limit its TIAH activities. It was Dr. Shannon who formalized this decision in a memorandum to the Public

147

Health Service Surgeon General and the HEW Secretary on October 4, 1966, stating that in his opinion, "total cardiac replacement is not a feasible program objective at the present time". Asked a decade later for the reaction of Mr. Fogarty and his colleagues in the Congress, the retired NIH director answered: "We explained it to them." Their acceptance of his scientific judgment indicates the measure of the Director's credibility on Capitol Hill.

What Dr. Shannon explained to them was the prevailing view of NIH leaders of that time. They argued that the real pay-off in heart, as in other biomedical research, lay not in making a massive effort to develop devices to replace diseased organs, but in finding out what caused them to become diseased in the first place. So little was known about the basic biological processes which lead to heart attack—that dangerous killer which so often strikes suddenly, and with terrible finality—and less than two percent of the Institute's budget was directed toward study of the heart attack event itself. It only made sense to turn more bioscientific attention and funding toward understanding heart attacks and thus, toward preventing them.

There were administrative considerations, too. The NIH leaders did not take kindly then, as they did not later in the War on Cancer disputes, to the idea of taking large amounts of research money and funneling them to profit making industrial firms through the targeted contract mechanism. Remembering the great resistance within the National Heart Institute and within the whole NIH, particularly among those concerned with extramural research grants, former NHI Director Knutti observes that indeed if he had been sitting in their chairs, he would have been opposed to TIAH too: "We believed that the grants program of the NIH was a program of, by and for the scientists. We had our study sections, we had careful review of every research project, they were studied at project site visits; it was, we thought, the best system that had been devised to give away money for scientific research."

More philosophically, but still in the realm of practicality, the NIH leaders sensed the awesome non-medical issues that might arise if they were successful in producing TIAH— the enormous cost in dollars and the difficult choices involved in selecting candidates for implantation. "As great as is the hope that cardiac replacement holds for the lives of a few", explained Dr. Donald Fredrickson, "so much greater is the insistence that better maintenance be found for the natural hearts and vessels of the multitude." As director of the National Heart Institute in 1968, he told the American College of Cardiology: "This is not to state that we should not build hearts or replace them. We will, but the pace and direction are determined only in part by ingenuity and skill; in part they must respond to the dictates of practicality."

As always, a minority dissented. Some clinical investigators argued they could learn more about the natural heart as they worked to develop its artificial replacement. They too, they said, were strong advocates of prevention. But when a 45 year old man's heart has degenerated from healthy muscle to weak leathery fibrous scar tissue, when the pumping chambers have shrunk to helpless size, then corrective surgery is impossible and all the drugs (chemotherapy) and all the tender loving care in the world will do little good. Admonishments about what might have been had the patient just stopped smoking and done more exercise might arouse anxiety and even do considerable harm. This man needs a new heart, and who is to say his medical needs should be ignored while the needs of others are attended?

As for the economic and social costs, it might be more practical to develop TIAH and eventually save the cost of years of expensive surgery and chemotherapy. Look how the development of the admittedly simpler and less costly pacemakers and valves in the 1950s had enhanced human well being and enabled hundreds of thousands of patients to lead normal productive lives. An investigator like Dr. Michael DeBakey has this perspective: before spectacles were ever invented, similar questions could have been asked. Should everyone wear them? Should only good people wear them? Would they be accepted? How are you going to manufacture them to make them readily available? "But once an idea proves feasible and effective," DeBakey argues, "it is bound to be accepted and society will find a way to make it available to everyone. Though we're still a long way from it, the same is going to be true about the artificial heart."

DeBakey had pioneered in the development of a family of assist devices to help the heart patient; indeed, he and his colleagues had described this approach in their early Advisory Group report. So it was that after the Shannon decision in 1966, the NHI's artificial heart program adopted four goals: emergency assist devices, temporary assist devices, an externally driven heart, and a totally implantable artificial heart. "We never thought it made sense simply to try to move the point of death from the street or office to the hospital," remembers Dr. Lowell T. Harmison, a bioengineer and physicist who joined the program as Dr. Hastings' deputy. "You need an emergency device to help the heart attack patient and get him to the point of medical evaluation and treatment. You need a temporary device to sustain him until his condition is stabilized or reversed. And you do not want merely to prolong life tied to a large console in the hospital without being able to offer the patient a permanent assist or total heart. Since heart disease is generally progressive, the more patients that are kept alive through drugs, surgery, or devices like pacemakers, the more that will eventually need total heart replacement."

Moving, then, toward the development of a series of therapeutic tools which the medical community might use for different cardiac patients—some so ill they could not lift a finger, others just in need of a device to tide them over a critical period—the artificial heart program scientists proceeded with several separate tasks.

Finding a material compatible with blood sounded simple. But it proved otherwise. When the inventories of industry yielded no such substance, and one after another had to be scrubbed, they began the search for a new biomaterial. This could be a promising silicone-like material (not yet discovered). Or it could be a material coated with heparin or another anticoagulant which prevents blood from clotting (it turned out that heparin works more effectively free in the bloodstream than attached to a surface). Or it could be a biological material coated with cells from the patient's own veins, a surface which would not have to be matched with his own body tissues (one of the most promising leads thus far).

Next, the innovators needed to develop a source of energy, preferably one which could last at least a decade. Devices powered by electricity or radio waves through the skin could of course be repaired or replaced more easily. But power packs would have to be carried about in an attache case or worn in a vest, and plugged into the wall when the patient reached home or office (and any wires permeating the skin posed the danger of infection or rejection). Although implantable power sources would be much more convenient and the patient using them would feel less dependent, they posed problems too. All generate heat, which has to be trapped or disseminated in the body. Batteries run out and have to be replaced, a biological fuel power cell causes complex blood chemical reactions, and a nuclear engine powered by a tiny plutonium capsule generates radiation with all its familiar potential effects on the user and others. Nonetheless, this avenue was explored through an at first cooperative arrangement with the Atomic Energy Commission, which later became a separate AEC (now Energy Research and Development Administration or ERDA) program directed toward TIAH alone. Three approaches to TIAH were involved:

An electric motor in the chest powered by a biological fuel cell or batteries planted in the abdomen.

151

A nuclear-powered heart that would not require recharging, with an energy source in the abdomen.

A miniaturized nuclear-powered heart completely implanted in the chest.

Then too, the scientists had to be concerned with the operation of the blood pump itself. How could it be controlled? How could it be made to work reliably—through a pulsing beat or a continuous pump flow? Above all, if such inventions were to be therapeutic and not merely experimental, the innovators needed to acquire a sound base of physiological and biological knowledge from animal studies. What effect, for instance, did the devices have on an animal's circulation, on its breathing, on its digestive system? On its brain and kidney and other vital organs?

The NHI continued to pursue these questions through grants to teams led by such clinical investigators as Dr. DeBakey, Dr. Adrian Kantrowitz, and Dr. Willem Kolff, while the artificial heart program used the contract mechanism systematically to organize the effort and to perform segments of the work, and held a series of contractor conferences to exchange ideas and stimulate interest. Their efforts in these days were complicated by the complex and not always happy marriage between engineers and medical scientists. The two disciplines, medicine the scientific art, and engineering with its underpinnings in the physical sciences, could not always fulfill each other's expectations. The NHI emphasis was naturally on the medical researcher and clinical investigator and their needs; the engineers, Dr. Harmison remembers, were often treated as "hardware kids", and many marriages between teams at hospital centers and industrial laboratories ended in divorce.

Still, they moved forward step by step, trying different materials, different power sources, and different combinations. With these, they hoped to evolve a way to control the artificial heart and fit it into the strange and wonderful biology of the human body.

152

Cardiowizardry: 1968 had been the year of the heart transplant. 101 were performed world wide, 54 in the United States*. Dr. Christiaan Barnard's first operations in Cape Town were, as Dr. Donald Fredrickson pointed out, "admittedly only mileposts along roads paved by hard work, commanding less attention." But they became a media event and the then-NHI director had to add, in his elegant prose, that such mileposts "have unparalleled power to grip the emotions of men separated by high mountains and deep oceans."

Such emotions were markedly tempered in most cardiovascular professional circles, especially in those where experienced clinical investigators had been proceeding cautiously and carefully toward Barnard's goal. There was a hint of scorn and perhaps of sour grapes at the South African surgeon's flamboyant publicity conscious style, and the prematurity of what one eminent medical research administrator called the "trick" he had performed. Medical politesse usually prevailed; seldom did anyone say such things publicly.

But both medical and lay commentators aired more serious concerns straightaway. They explained that the human body fights to reject foreign natural organs in the same way it fights infections. A heart transplant patient can suffer acute or chronic rejection, and if he is given too many immunosuppressive drugs to counteract this rejection, he may fall victim to severe infections like pneumonia. Such problems are many times more severe in heart than in kidney transplant patients because unlike the kidney, the heart can never rest. It must work constantly, second by second, minute by minute, or the patient will die. The skilled hand of the cardiovascular surgeon had outstripped the basic scientist's knowledge of immunology.

---

*Two of the 101 and one of the 54 had survived as of January 1, 1976, according to the American College of Surgeons/NIH Organ Transplant Registry. Altogether, 64 transplant teams in 22 countries have done 296 heart transplant operations; 52 recipients survive.

By 1969 such fears had been confirmed; too few heart transplant patients survived for too short periods of time, and the experts acquired little clear evidence as to why those who did survive lived on. Enthusiasm cooled; the number of transplants world-wide dropped to 47 in 1969 (two survive), 34 of them in the United States (one survives), and to 17 worldwide in 1970, 16 of them in the United States (all three survivors live in the United States). This slowdown began to be called a moratorium.

Dr. Peter Frommer, who now heads the Cardiovascular Devices Branch (once the artificial heart program), points out that there are two sorts of medical moratoria here. The government can stop funding research which, for some reason, it deems unworthy of public support; for such decisions NIH relies heavily on peer review study section advice. Or the profession can impose a moratorium on an experimental procedure itself, as it clearly did in the case of heart transplantation. No heart transplant has ever been performed at NIH's Clinical Center. Although the NHLI has funded some of the major basic and clinical research in the field, its role has been that of monitor and evaluator, but not of leader. Reacting at the end of 1968 when interest in the transplant effort was still at its height, it circumspectly appointed an Ad Hoc Task Force on Cardiac Replacement to examine a number of broad questions regarding cardiac replacement, including artificial hearts and assist devices, for people under 65.

In an intriguing, well-documented study*, Renée C. Fox, a sociologist, and Judith P. Swazey, a biologist and scientific historian, analyze what they call "the courage to fail ethos". They report that the moratorium on heart transplants was first

---

* *The Courage to Fail: A Social View of Organ Transplants and Dialysis,* by Renée C. Fox and Judith P. Swazey, The University of Chicago Press, 1974. I am indebted to their study especially for its accounts of the Montreal Moratorium and also for their detailed chapter on the artificial heart implant in Houston.

officially announced at the Montreal Heart Insitute in January, 1969. At this Institute, founded in the conviction that French Canadians should enjoy the finest possible cardiovascular facilities and share the prestige of innovation, Dr. Pierre Grondin and his surgical team had performed nine transplants. Dr. Grondin had trained with Doctors DeBakey and Denton A. Cooley in Houston, and emulated their can-do attitude and their pursuit of excellence. But as his nine patients fell prey to rejection or massive infection, and as other transplant surgeons began to report similar results, the Institute found the courage to fail, and formally announced its decision. National pride, the intense desire to save life, the pioneering, gutsy, indefatigable, fiercely competitive work oriented character of the closely bound community of transplant surgeons made the decision a difficult one. But the arguments for discontinuing were stronger than the reach for extreme measures, and the heart transplant was formally removed from the hospital's armamentarium.

Enthusiasm dimmed among other hospital teams as well. As the public read about discouraging results, the number of operations began to diminish; some teams performed one or two, then jumped off the bandwagon. The slowdown resulted in a fall in the supply of heart donors and helped lead to the famous, or infamous, episode of the artificial heart implant. Turning, the spotlight fell on Texas, and a first, but not a proud moment in medical history, one marked by melodrama, stealth and a tangled web of relations between two surgical giants and their subordinates.

These are the facts:* on April 4, 1969 at St. Luke's Episcopal Hospital in Houston, Dr. Denton Cooley implanted the device—a biventricular pump driven by a large console outside the body—in the chest of a 47 year old man named Haskell Karp. The implant was actually the second stage of a three-stage procedure. Dr. Cooley first attempted a ventriculoplasty, sometimes called a wedge excision or resection.

*See *Karp v. Cooley,* 493 F2d 408 (1974).

When that proved unsuccessful, the surgeon implanted the mechanical heart and it sustained the patient for about 64 hours until a donor heart became available. (After an emotionally charged television plea by Mrs. Karp, a donor arrived in an air-ambulance from Massachusetts.) The artificial heart was removed from Haskell Karp's chest, the donor's heart was implanted on the morning of April 7. Karp died at 4:10 p.m. on April 8, 1969, some 32 hours later, of pneumonia and renal or kidney failure.

The National Heart Institute was involved in this episode only because the device in question had, in fact, been developed at the Baylor-Rice University artificial heart program funded by NHI through its principal investigator, Dr. Michael DeBakey. DeBakey did not know about the Karp implantation, and did not feel that the machine's technical or physiological problems had been solved or that it had been sufficiently tested in animals. The mechanical pump had been covertly removed without his permission from the Baylor laboratory, where it had been built in an atmosphere of great secrecy, under the direction of Dr. Domingo S. Liotta, a DeBakey research assistant (a surgeon apparently impatient to move from animal experimentation to clinical use and flattered when one of his heroes, Dr. Cooley, suggested they work together on an artificial heart.) The large console which powered the pump was duplicated by its designer, an engineer in the NHI-funded program, in his private garage—also at Liotta's request for Dr. Cooley, and at Cooley's expense—and delivered to St. Luke's with a note that it was for animal experimentation only.

A series of probes started the day after the artificial device implant, as the news broke and various officials tried to determine exactly what had happened and why. Baylor University itself conducted several inquiries. From Washington, the National Heart Institute's director, Dr. Theodore Cooper, asked for and got verification that the artificial heart in question had been developed with NHI funds. No protocol for clinical implantation had been submitted to

Baylor's research committee; the heart had been used clinically without NHI peer review and approval, and the Public Health Service guidelines for human experimentation had not been followed. Cooper pointedly asked what stringent measures were being taken to insure that NHI and Baylor protocols would be followed in the future.

Baylor proposed such new regulations; subsequently Dr. Cooley refused to sign a statement agreeing to abide by them and resigned from the medical school faculty. Later he was to speak of the sore need for the device in question and call its first implantation his patriotic duty. Dr. Liotta was discharged from the Baylor-Rice artificial heart program. About a year later, Mrs. Haskell Karp filed a $4 million medical malpractice suit against St. Luke's, Doctors Cooley and Liotta and the engineer who had worked with them during the implant, Sam Calvin, claiming that her husband had been the victim of human experimentation.

Among other wrongs, she asserted that consent to the operation was fraudulently obtained, and that the defendants were negligent in performing the corrective surgery and implanting the artificial heart. But she could not mobilize the testimony she needed and the federal trial judge in southern Texas directed a verdict against her. This decision was affirmed on appeal in April of 1974 by the U.S. Circuit Court of Appeals in New Orleans.*

Not a very pretty story. But it did force attention on the need to create an artificial heart which would not tie its recipient to a bedside console for life. NHI's artificial heart program scientists had in fact proceeded in this direction. At first, they had searched for such separate parts of TIAH and the family of assist devices as biomaterials and an energy

---

*In *The Courage to Fail,* Rénee Fox and Judith Swazey describe the medical fraternity's unwillingness to speak out and discipline a fellow member, and also the reluctance of the technicians and engineers to challenge a physician-superior.

source. In the spring of 1969, they began to emphasize putting the various parts together, first in an implantable left heart assist (LVAD) and then in a completely implantable device which could be tested in animals. They called this their "saltation", or leaping ahead effort.

Heart transplants had raised some puzzling questions about the rights of both donors and recipients.* Now the Karp case focused attention on questions which applied to transplants and mechanical hearts as well:

Had the procedure or device been adequately tested in animals? At what point was it ready for clinical use? Had new scientific complexities and concepts of individual rights obsoleted the surgical pioneer who plunged ahead to help his hopelessly ill patient in a lets-get-the-job-done fashion? Had the patient's voluntary and informed consent been obtained? Did the benefits outweigh the suffering and risk and costs involved? How about distributive justice—did it make sense, was it just, to fly a terminally ill donor across the country to give her heart to another terminally ill patient when it may have benefited someone nearby more?

The NHI had never completely ignored such questions. Its first artificial heart evaluation, done under contract in 1966, had summarized in technical terms the need to produce a device which would meet the recipient's social and psychological as well as medical needs, help restore and rehabilitate him, and improve the quality of his life. Its second evaluation, the Ad Hoc Task Force report *Cardiac Replacement**, produced in the fall of 1969, expanded on these themes with regard to heart transplants as well as artificial hearts.

---

*The Uniform Anatomical Gift Act, adopted now by all the states, provides safeguards for donor and donee (but leaves the definition of when death occurs to individual state law).

**"Cardiac Replacement: Medical, Ethical, Psychological and Economic Implications", A Report by Ad Hoc Task Force on Cardiac Replacement, National Heart Institute, (Government Printing Office, Washington) October 1969.

The task force reported that progress had been made on some of the issues involved. It pointed out that the Nazi atrocities in human experimentation had led to the adoption, after the War, of the Nuremberg Code, which enunciated such requirements as truly voluntary consent of the subject to experimentation; protection of the subject against mental and physical harm; the likelihood of fruitful results unprocurable by other means; care that risk taken does not exceed the humanitarian importance of the problem, and avoidance of unnecessary injury.

The Code principles were reaffirmed by the World Medical Association meeting in Helsinki in 1964, which also said that the doctor can combine clinical research with patient care only to the extent that it is justified by its therapeutic value to the patient, and that it is the doctor's duty to remain the protector of the life and health of all research subjects. When it opened its doors, NIH's Clinical Center had published guidelines involving informed consent and peer review to make certain that potential risks did not outweigh potential benefits.* The Kefauver-Harris amendments to the Food Drug, and Cosmetics Act of 1962 had restimulated NIH concern and after considerable study, in 1966 the guidelines were extended to cover the U.S. Public Health Service's extramural grants and awards. In 1971 these principles were made generally applicable to all HEW extramural activities involving human subjects.

Except for the unresolved problem of finding a generally acceptable medical definition of death, *Cardiac Replacement*

---

*NIH Director Donald Fredrickson, who participated in the small group which put the guidelines together, remembers his "increased awareness" that in their innocence, he and his medical research colleagues had quite honestly felt they had the right to seek knowledge for the good of society. As they worked with lawyers to develop the new standards they realized the preeminence of the rights of individual patients to consent to and benefit from their participation in medical research.

noted, transplantation did not seem to raise problems for the Protestant, Catholic or Jewish faiths. But it added that Congress, the scientific community, and the general public had yet to face difficult decisions: the allocation of health funds between prevention and treatment; the need to draw a line between prolonging life and prolonging the process of dying; the need to weigh the cost of cardiac replacement against other medical and social needs; the financing of individual replacements.

In Congress, Senator Walter Mondale of Minnesota had first tried to focus attention on such questions when he proposed a National Commission on Health, Science and Society in 1968. His proposal, he said, was a "measly little study commission to look at some very profound technological breakthroughs which could revolutionize human society." Nonetheless, it ran into unexpected opposition among some members of the scientific community, in whom he sensed "an almost psychopathic objection to the public process," a fear that if the public got involved it would be anti-science, hostile and unsupportive. "They bootlegged Christiaan Barnard in here to tell us . . . 'You will have a politician in every surgical room'," Mondale was to say later about the hearings before Senator Fred Harris' Government Operations Subcommittee on his proposal (S.J. Res. 145). "They got Dr. (Arthur) Kornberg in here, who is a great scientist and . . . he asked us, 'Why are you wasting my time here?'"

Reintroducing his proposal (as S.J. Res. 75) in 1971, Mondale warned, "We can ill afford to wait until the crush of events forces us to make hasty and often ill-considered decisions". This time there was some change in attitude; scientists had begun to realize the proposal called not for a regulatory, but for an advisory commission to conduct a series of studies. The advent not only of transplants and artificial organs but also of rapid advances in the possibilities of genetic engineering and behavior modification confronted an in-

160

creasing awareness of the rights of the human subjects. The realization grew that the public faced what Herbert Jasper, a Mondale staffer, called some pretty "hairy problems"— problems in which new forms of life could be created and some existing forms changed or sustained indefinitely. More came to agree with Mondale that "this cannot be—and should not be a private process. The public stake is too great". Although HEW's Assistant Secretary for Health testified against the resolution, NIH Director Robert Marston spoke up during hearings before the Senate Health Subcommittee, to say his agency supported the commission idea; questions of such magnitude could not be held within the scientific community. S.J. Res. 75 passed the Senate, but did not get anywhere in the House.

Now a new set of circumstances focused on that always important consideration—money. On November 4, 1971, Shep Glazer, an official of the National Association of Patients on Hemodialysis was dialyzed by his wife (with a physician present at the Committee Counsel's request) before the House Ways and Means Committee considering different national health insurance proposals. A year later, after continued lobbying by patients and their advocates, but with little public discussion and no committee consideration, the Congress extended the Medicare program to cover end-stage renal patients under 65. In its first year (1973-74) the program was to cost $240 million for some 13,000 patients entitled to kidney dialysis or transplants. The government estimates it will cost an annual $1 billion for 50,000-60,000 patients by 1984.

The Ethics Report; deemphasis: By 1972 the NHI scientists' saltation or leaping ahead effort was going well. In that year, its first cardiac assist device, a capillary oxygenator, reached the stage of limited clinical trial, and this temporary device for respiratory support was used during open heart surgery at several hospitals. In that year, the program scientists successfully tested a totally implantable nuclear powered heart

161

in calves, and applied for a patent for it.* In that year, too, the National Heart, Blood Vessel, Lung and Blood Act became law. The Institute's budget was due to expand. Its horizons seemed at the moment, limitless.

Still, the feeling grew that society had been caught unprepared by the advent of heroic technologies like the transplants. Ironically, just as the scientists began to move toward TIAH, the impossible questions—reflecting the *Zeitgeist* of the 1970s, but really present from the beginning—began to catch up with it. Around the National Heart and Lung Institute more and more people asked "If we had the total heart, would we know what to do with it?" And, "would it be worth the hundreds of millions it would cost to develop it?"

So it was, that in the summer of 1972, NHLI Director Theodore Cooper convened a panel composed of three doctors (an internist, cardiologist and psychiatrist), two lawyers, two economists, a sociologist, political scientist and a priest-ethicist, and chaired by Harold P. Green, Professor of Law at George Washington University. By the following June, it was to assess the economic, ethical, legal, medical, psychiatric and social implications of the totally implantable heart.

Most often, non-expert politicians or administrators convene expert groups to advise them on specific questions; with the technical facts in hand, they feel they can then make informed political judgments. Here, on the contrary, the technically competent NHLI had approved a group composed largely of laymen; outside of the three physicians, they knew little about the technical matter at hand, but had a great deal of knowledge which might be brought to bear on its implications for the body politic. The Institute's Constance F. Row (who had assisted Senator Mondale during the hearings on his first study commission proposal) and Deputy Director Robert Ringler told the panel that what Institute officials wanted was

---

*On November 18, 1975, Patent 3919722 was issued to Lowell T. Harmison and assigned to the U.S. Government as represented by the Secretary of the Department of Health, Education and Welfare.

not a simple neutral technology assessment of the consequences of TIAH, but an idea of what surprises might be in store for them, in getting from here to there. When alternative models or sets of standards would lead to importantly different implications, their recommendations would be welcome.

"Most government advisory committees and panels look at a problem, describe it as they would in an article in *Scientific American*, and say 'Oh My!' ", observed one of the panelists later. "We were supposed to say more than 'Oh My!' ". That they did. Although most felt their charge ambiguous, and several submitted detailed minority views on different aspects, as a group they tackled vigorously and seriously the bioethical issues of distributive justice, social cost and public safety. Familiarity sometimes breeds contempt. In this case, it bred acceptance, and some definite doubts. As the panelists went about their job, they grew less and less in awe of TIAH and came to think of its impact as similar to that of other major medical innovations. They came to think of their report as a human impact statement, and of their forum as a means for gaining societal informed consent to a form of medical experimentation and treatment.

Nevertheless, they surely recognized TIAH's significance, and urged that every effort be made to engage the public in a dialogue as to its potential impact. Wondering whether the artificial development of this central organ "might not only place technology in man's bosom, but place man more deeply in the bosom of technology,"* they asked what other natural

---

*See "The Totally Implantable Artificial Heart: Legal, Social, Ethical, Medical, Economic, Psychological Implications," A Report of the Artificial Heart Assessment Panel of the National Heart and Lung Institute, HEW Publication 74-191, June 1973. Two Hastings Center Reports have analyzed the Panel's work: "The Totally Implantable Artificial Heart" by Albert R. Jonsen, November 1973, and "The Case of the Artificial Heart Panel," by Morris Bernard Kaplan, October 1975, published by the Institute of Society, Ethics and the Life Sciences.

parts of the body would be replaced by a machine in the future? The brain? The stomach? The sex organs? Would the recipient regard himself and would others regard him as more, or less human? What would his dependence on a machine mean? How escape the criticism leveled at other technologies that TIAH would treat life as an end in itself whatever that life's nature and quality? How to balance more relatively normal productive years against the possibility of a more painful, lingering death from cancer or stroke, particularly among the aged?

Cautiously, the panelists recommended that TIAH's development should proceed, for it would be useful and important therapy, if all the expectations of its sponsors were realized. But its development should be carefully monitored by a broadly constituted group and its scope and content periodically reconsidered and balanced with that of heart disease prevention and other treatment programs. Of special interest to NIHers: the program's success might establish an important precedent for the development of goal-directed, technologically sophisticated solutions to public health problems.

Who would get TIAH? At whose expense and at what economic and social cost to the whole society? The question of distributive justice dominated the panel's report. The majority recommended careful planning to minimize the possibility that the artificial heart would be in short supply. But if it were necessary, candidates should be selected by physicians and medical institutions, according to medical criteria. If demand exceeded supply, social worth criteria should not be used; patients should be chosen randomly. In other words, with the choice between a Secretary of State, a coal miner, a taxi driver, a business executive and a waitress, all of whom met the medical criteria, the recipient should be chosen by lot.

If social worth, or unworth should not bar TIAH, neither should cost. Most panelists felt that the artificial heart's expense would make financing by the patient impossible, unless it were covered by insurance, government or private. Particularly in view of the substantial public funds used in

164

development, availability should not be limited by ability to pay.

And there was a newer, more ominous cost which had to be considered. In view of the risks to the families and associates of recipients, and to the public and the environment, the nuclear powered heart should not be implanted in human beings until it had been scientifically determined through animal tests that it could be used without significant risk. Such testing could proceed in animals, and if it proved successful, the heart could be tested in a limited number of patients.

The panel was attracted to the idea of a reliable, compact, long-lived nuclear powered heart. But here it had been discouraged by expert testimony, not so much about the considerable long range effect of radiation on recipients, all of whom would be seriously ill with heart disease without TIAH, but about the slight but significant effect on others. It might mean genetic damage; it might create or enhance the danger of leukemia or some other type of cancer for spouses sleeping in the same bed. One scientist testified he would not feel comfortable seated between two recipients on an airplane. Quite clearly, general use of the device would add in a statistically trivial way to the background of radiation in the atmosphere—causing perhaps 1 excess case of cancer against 7,200 which occur spontaneously.

"What we really told them was to cool it," concludes panelist Dr. Albert R. Jonsen, Professor of Bioethics at the University of California School of Medicine. Cool it they did, but it is hard to find a consensus among NHLI officials and others prominently involved as to the exact extent of the panel's influence. These range all the way from the medical scientists who pooh-pooh it, saying that ethics is too dangerous a subject to be left to the ethicists (and no medical discovery would ever be made if it had to await panel decisions), to those who credit the panel with the subsequent shift of emphasis away from a nuclear system to battery and biological fuel system research and toward the less ambitious Left Ventricular Assist Device (LVAD).

Former NHLI Director, now Assistant HEW Secretary Dr. Theodore Cooper, who should know, feels that through thoughtful, vigorous and open discussion the panel illuminated the issues involved, and that this did indeed have its effect on the Institute and its advisory council.

One finding had a special effect, Cooper reports. The NHLI leaders looked hard at the pool of patients that the panel reported would be candidates for the artificial heart. Dramatic surgical advances since 1969 in coronary artery and congenital heart disease, and improvement in artificial valves, had increased the number of these patients to 16,750-50,300 and probably closer to the higher estimate, instead of the 11,736-32,168 estimated by *Cardiac Replacement* in 1969 (a number which included heart transplant candidates but excluded those over 65, while the panel included patients up to the age of 75.) They looked hard at the cost of its development (from $100 million to over $1 billion) and at its cost to individual patients and insurors ($15,000 to $25,000 per patient*). They looked hard at the Institute's resources and its growing inability to meet all the different demands the new 1972 law had made of it. They were skeptical of the imminence of real breakthroughs in artificial heart technology. Cooper reports he spent a great deal of time assessing the unfolding of the technology involved—on questions of biomaterials for example—and concluded that "there was not too much new out there to seed."

In the end, the artificial heart program, which had been reshuffled and renamed several times and had seen a succession of helmsmen after the untimely death of Dr. Frank Hastings, became a small part of the NHLI's Cardiovascular Devices Branch. In early 1976, branch chief Dr. Peter Frommer estimated that about 5 percent of his $12.9 million devices budget, covering both grants and contracts, went to the

---

*The National Academy of Sciences' Institute of Medicine estimated in 1973 that the national resource cost of treating end-stage heart disease by implanting an artificial heart would range from slightly less than $600 million to slightly more than $1.75 billion a year.

development of TIAH, 25 percent to LVAD and 70 percent to the development of components like biomaterials which could be used for both. ERDA (the Energy Research and Development Administration, successor to the AEC research program) was still conducting a $3.5 million a year program geared to the development of a nuclear powered heart. But it looked as though the Office of Management and Budget would succeed in cutting it out after several tries, despite the bedazzlement of legislators like Senator Joseph M. Montoya, the Joint Atomic Energy Committee's Legislation Subcommittee Chairman, who commented during 1975 hearings that he thought artificial heart research "really sheds considerable credit on atomic energy research because this is one of the spin-offs of that research. It really glamorizes the atomic energy research program and gives it greater attraction so far as the people are concerned even among those who are critical of atomic energy research."

Heart transplants have not stopped altogether; in fact, the outstanding remaining transplant team, led by Dr. Norman Shumway at Stanford University Medical Center, continues to make progress. Under a $525,000 three-year NHLI grant, this team's postoperative three month survival rates had risen to 85-90 percent and almost half of their carefully selected patients are surviving for a year. In experienced able hands, extraordinarily sensitive to the scientific problems of rejection and able to respond to them very early, transplantation can continue. But it is, as NHLI Director Dr. Robert Levy puts it, investigational.

The Cardiovascular Devices Branch program focuses now on the development of a left ventricular assist device as a logical next step, since it is almost always the heart's left ventricle which fails. In 1975, the Branch announced approval of human clinical trials for the LVAD in selected patients difficult to wean from the heart-lung machine. This was an assist device powered by a large external console; far from replacing the heart, it takes over a fraction of the work for its main pumping chamber for a few weeks at a time. The

167

Associated Press news story that went out across the country said that the LVAD implants at Houston (by Dr. John C. Norman of the Texas Heart Institute) and at Boston (by Dr. William F. Bernhard of Children's Hospital Medical Center) marked a significant milestone toward the goal of artificial heart implants. It added that cardiologists believe that the artificial heart, when perfected, will be the overwhelming choice of patients because they will be more reliable than live heart transplants, which the body tries to reject as a foreign substance, and will give rise to fewer ethical and legal problems.

As 1976 began, there was no longer any doubt that the application of a technology like the artificial heart raised questions beyond the limits of scientific expertise; on the contrary, there had been an explosion of public interest in these questions, official and non-official. The substance of Senator Mondale's original study proposal had been included as a minor part of the mandate of the National Commission for the Protection of Human Subjects, despite Mondale's urging that the study required the concentrated attention of a separate commission. The Commission had been created by Congress (under Title II of the 1974 Research Service Award Act) as a result chiefly of pressures from two diverse sources—civil rights groups, stirred by violations of the rights of deprived and institutionalized human subjects, and anti-abortionists concerned with the rights of the unborn—and its work had centered on their specific immediate concerns. It met the four month deadline to recommend guidelines for the conduct of foetal research (a foetus scheduled to be aborted had the same rights as a foetus to be carried to term) and then went on to formulate standards for research on prisoners, children and the institutionalized mentally infirm. Mondale's more general ethics proposal has been largely relegated to a "Delphi Study," a conference by mail, in which 125 participants (ethicists, lawyers, physicians, social and physical scientists) attempt to reach conclusions about the implications of such subjects as

168

reproductive engineering, the use of data banks and mechanisms which extend life.

When it came to ethics questions, the Disease of the Month Club had turned into the Commission of the Month Club. The law already provided that when it had completed its work, the National Commission for the Protection of Human Subjects would go out of business and a new National Advisory Council would take its place. But, during the past year Senator Edward Kennedy introduced two proposals to create new Commissions: a permanent independent Commission for the Protection of Human Subjects broadening the present commission's jurisdiction to the whole government, including the C.I.A. and F.B.I.; and with Senator Gary Hart, a National Health Research and Development Advisory Commission financed by a cigarette tax based on nicotine content, and empowered to oversee, evaluate and recommend priorities for all federal health research.

Congress' Office of Technology Assessment had established an Advisory Panel on Biomedical Research and Medical Technology, chaired by Duke University Medical Center's Dr. Eugene A. Stead and including Dr. Lewis Thomas, the physician-scientist-poet who has described devices like TIAH as half way technologies. This group's task was to consider whether proof of efficacy and safety should be legally required of costly new medical technologies and procedures before they are put into general use, as it is before new drugs can be used. The National Academy of Sciences' Institute of Medicine had set up an Advisory Committee on Social Ethics and Health under a three year Andrew W. Mellon Foundation grant. It may have been that Senator Mondale was right—the Congress should have created the Commission he proposed in the first place.

Symposia, conferences, courses and seminars addressing medical ethics abound; forty-seven medical schools offer elective bioethics courses. An increasing number of Americans are realizing that the enormous benefits conferred by modern medicine are no longer, as the experts say, inestimable. Each benefit must be balanced not only against alternative benefits, but also against the complex psychological, social, financial and environmental costs and risks involved. How to do this remains a formidable challenge. Money alone is not an acceptable measurement for most Americans when human lives are so intimately involved. Other human values must be weighed in a framework of social cost-benefit analysis as yet undefined. If the scientists produced a perfect, long lasting artificial heart, completely reliable, efficient and safe, which would offer a decade of productive life to you or to me, many feel the government would opt for it, no matter how many dollars were involved.

When is a "lag" between bench and bedside too long? Too short? Just right? In a paper prepared for the President's Biomedical Research Panel, Dr. Julius Comroe, Jr. explores these questions and concludes that lags—the number of years between initial discovery and its effective clinical application— are too short when their application becomes widespread before limitations and risks are fully known; they are too long when all the necessary knowledge is at hand but it is not applied to clinical medicine or surgery; they can be just right even though the lag is long in years when many completely unforeseen discoveries are needed for the final clinical advance.

Some say Dr. James Shannon showed exquisite scientific taste in first containing the search for TIAH a decade ago; they would deny any undue delay in its development. Some challenge the Shannon decision—but it still stands at NIH, reinforced a hundredfold by the impossible decisions. Asked recently what he would do if NHLI director Robert Levy came to him and said "We have an artificial heart," the man who now fills Shannon's shoes, Dr. Donald Fredrickson, said he would "not exactly cry out with joy. It is a very costly temporary solution to heart disease and not an appropriate piece of technology for today." Only time can assess this judgment. Only time will tell how to characterize the "lag" in TIAH—as too long, too short, or just right.

170

9.   The Oncoming Waves

"We explained it to them", former NIH Director Dr. James Shannon answered, when asked how his decision to contain artificial heart research had affected its Congressional advocates. A decade later, it is doubtful that he or any other NIH Director could report such a feat so simply and so crisply. There are too many of "them", and with health research just a part of the large "H" enterprise, "we" no longer can refer to a compact group in and around NIH.

One finds it difficult to select a single man or woman personifying any part of the complex health politics picture. Of the health leaders on Capitol Hill, of course, Senator Edward M. Kennedy is most familiar to the public and as the active Chairman of the Senate Labor and Public Welfare Committee's Health Subcommittee, he has astutely dramatized issue after issue. But more than most legislators he is a media superstar spread out over a whole panopoly of other issues, from Viet Nam refugees to federal election laws. And unlike the man who once held his job, former Senator Lister Hill, he does not also chair the Health Appropriations Subcommittee. It is that subcommittee, now commandingly led by Senator Warren G. Magnuson, which apportions monies to health programs. Nor, although Kennedy has helped lay the groundwork through planning and manpower laws, do his committee assignments give him direct access to the over-

arching issue of shaping national health insurance programs which will largely determine how the fruits of medical research are delivered. That is the job of the Senate Finance Committee, chaired by Senator Russell B. Long.

Many, many Senators and Congressmen now work to leave their thumbprints on the $118 billion health care industry. Of all of them, perhaps Chairman Paul G. Rogers of the House Subcommittee on Health and the Environment emerges as the most significant. Energetic, well-informed, skillful at Congressional give and take and bolstered by over twenty years of seniority, he has worked to expand his jurisdiction over health matters. Although the health appropriations process is now presided over by Pennsylvania's Representative Daniel J. Flood, Rogers has tried to reach out for the national health insurance issue, previously the undisputed turf of the Ways and Means Committee. After the political demise of former Chairman Wilbur D. Mills, Rogers scheduled repeated national health insurance hearings, sometimes duplicating those of Ways and Means Health Subcommittee Chairman Dan Rostenkowski.

On television talk shows and in news magazines, enthusiastic commentators have referred to the soft-spoken and impeccably dressed Congressman from West Palm Beach as "Mr. Health", and his office biographical handout claims that "virtually every major law in the area of health bears the Rogers mark". Realistically, however, like other key members of the lower house, Rogers remains primarily an insiders' figure, the man for the ever increasing tribe of health lobbyists to see. As such, Paul Rogers is an ally of the NIHers, but not their agent—by no means willing to grant their every request as was the Congressman with whom he is increasingly compared, the late John Fogarty. Recalling the difficult days when very hard line Nixonians had almost, he thought, made up their minds "to do away with NIH, even to break it up or destroy it", Rogers speaks of Congressional determination to gain support

172

and a greater measure of stability for that agency; after the first Alumni Reunion, he gave a platform to eminent NIHers who extolled their agency and warned against letting it go downhill. He agrees that an excellent NIH is essential to continued research progress. Still, like most of his colleagues, he speaks of the necessity for health cost savings and for accountability— obtaining tangible results for government dollars invested in health research. In measures like research training, as we have seen, he comes off more on the side of the NIHers than do Senators such as Edward Kennedy, but he, too, demanded that trainees repay the government according to a stiff formula.

Is there a new Dr. Shannon? Or Mary Lasker? Out in Bethesda, NIH Director Dr. Donald S. Fredrickson is fast establishing himself as a prestigious biomedical leader, and Paul Rogers has taken pains to get to know him and bring his subcommittee and staff out for a campus tour. But in the Republican management-minded scheme of things, the health research enterprise is only one of six H agencies; it is the HEW Assistant Secretary for Health, Dr. Theodore Cooper, who speaks, or tries to speak, for the health team in the highest councils of government. NIHers tend to regard him as one of themselves: Does he not still live on the campus, and is he not an architect of the modern broad approach to heart disease research, which, according to mortality statistics, is beginning to pay off?

As Congressman Paul Rogers points out, however, the political life span of contemporary Assistant Secretaries is short. What's more, the health decision making power may be vested not in them, or their knowledgeable program managers, but in middle level Office of Management and Budget bureaucrats (who are part management specialists and part political strategists for the President). Although the feisty, self-contained, hard-working Ted Cooper—a physician short in stature but not in ability, a Democrat in a Republican Administration—commands wide respect on and off Capitol

173

Hill, he has to walk on eggs trying to formulate health policy, competing within the Department and with OMB officials first for the Secretarial and then for the Presidential ear.

Mary Lasker is still very much around, a member of the Cancer Advisory Board and health activist on many pro bono issues. A woman born at the turn of the century, she is reluctant now to discuss the past accomplishments of the Lasker lobby, preferring to press forward, insisting we are not moving fast enough or with enough sense of urgency, or spending enough on health research. But if any non-government figure has come to serve as a strategic broker between the biomedical scientists and the politicians who shape health policy, it is Benno C. Schmidt, the big bushy eyebrowed Republican financier out of Texas and New York who became active in national health politics during the War on Cancer days. Suave, self-assured, pragmatic, a man obviously used to presiding at most of the meetings he attends, he chairs the President's Cancer Panel and served during its fifteen months activity in 1975 and 1976 as an influential member of the President's Biomedical Research Panel as well.* Chauffered around Washington in a long black limousine, he makes good use of his contacts in high places in the cause, first of cancer, but of other health research as well— explaining a point of view he has come to understand: "You cannot target unless you have an adequate science base; I wish we had more we could target".

Who can speak for the medical scientists without whom research could not be accomplished? Who can interpret the biomedical scientists' search for truth to the scientifically unlettered who pay the bills and may reap the benefits? Here we can turn to Dr. Lewis Thomas, accomplished prose stylist and

---

*This 7-member panel was mandated by the Congress under the Cancer Act Amendments of 1974. It was directed to study the policy issues confronting health research and make recommendations for future work and organization of the health research agencies. The panel in turn appointed clusters or task forces composed of distinguished scientists.

essayist*, *physician, pathologist, virologist, former dean, president of New York Memorial Sloan-Kettering Cancer Center, and recipient for many years of NHLI grant support for the study of rheumatic fever (and of other NIH support as well). During the work of the President's Biomedical Research Panel, he chaired "The Overview Cluster", a macro-micro committee which synthesized the work of eleven different other clusters representing fields like immunology or biochemistry, and composed of some of the nation's most distinguished scientists.*

Sixty-two now, in, as he puts it, "his stocking feet", Dr. Thomas looks at the place of bioscience in medicine and finds it good. The tears of the cancer or heart attack victim, or the despair of the ghetto mother waiting at night in the city hospital emergency room, seem far away when you talk to this horn-rimmed, thoughtful, likeable physician. He is an optimist. When his father practiced medicine in Flushing there was not so much doctors could do for their patients, though they found great satisfaction in useful service. Every family had four or five members cut down in their prime by lobar pneumonia or tuberculosis. Today, thanks to the biological revolution which brought modern immunization and antibiotics, and thanks too to improved sanitation, nutrition and housing, we are in danger of becoming a nation of healthy hypochondriacs—living to 72, enjoying a mortality rate of 1 percent (pretty good since you have to die anyway), but jogging and fussing so hard to stay healthy, we live scared. We want to enjoy long, pain free lives until the moment when all our parts collapse simultaneously, like Oliver Wendell Holmes' Deacon's Masterpiece, "the wonderful one-hoss shay".

Dr. Thomas has been on so many advisory councils and committees that he has been obliged, he says, to do a certain

---

*His collection of essays, *The Lives of a Cell: Notes of a Biology Watcher (Viking Press, 1974)* won a National Book Award in the arts and letters, not the science category, a fact which pleased him greatly.

amount of thinking about public policy. Here again, he is an optimist. Like most of his fellow biomedical scientists, he stresses the slow, stepwise extension of what came before: breakthroughs are not revelations, they are based on solid stores of information accumulated over long years in which scientists grappled with small, humble questions. Look at the recent explosion of knowledge documented in the individual cluster reports. The Biochemistry, Molecular Genetics and Cell Biology group headed by Nobelist Dr. George E. Palade, explained that the work of the last years has not generated more knowledge about critical health problems because it has been attempting to understand the components of the cell— from genome to membrane—their organization and basic chemical reactions. Only now does the prerequisite body of information begin to approach a level from which the investigation of regulatory mechanisms can start.

Dr. Thomas pleads for patience: a quarter of a century from now if we can keep fresh young minds coming into the research system, he is sure the major chronic illnesses like cardiovascular disease will be coming under control; we will be able to prevent hardening of the arteries; even to reverse it. It would be a mistake now to try to centralize and systematize our efforts further; the movement and strength of science depends on the imagination and intuition in the heads of investigators in their laboratories or on their hospital wards. Their search will lead not to the halfway technology measures which must be taken to compensate for the destructive effects of disease, but to the truly high technologies like the polio vaccine which aim directly at the cause of a disease so that it can be terminated, reversed or prevented outright.

So the issue is joined: the scientists point to past progress and future expectations and ask for patience. Elected officials, representing voters, in whose breasts the hope for immortality or at least a pain-free old age springs eternal, ask for accountability or cures and preventives at a faster pace, in

176

return for public money. NIH, the government's chief health research agency, stands in the middle.

The year that followed the first Alumni Reunion brought a modicum of peace to the National Institutes of Health campus. The malaise seemed to have lifted; the age of Watergate was over, and with it had passed what Paul Rogers called "the difficult days"—the days in which the hardline Nixonians had tried to retaliate for lack of political support among the scientists and academicians, and, as some saw it, to bring the intellectuals to heel. Though they were not exactly dancing on their well kept lawns, the NIHers felt less estranged than they had in many a year.

At least they had emerged from limbo. Downtown, they had—temporarily—some friends in court. As Assistant Secretary for Health, Dr. Theodore Cooper had replaced Dr. Charles Edwards, a silver haired, smoothly mannered executive and surgeon who had condescendingly warned NIHers that they could not live in happy isolation from budget realities and must learn to fit into their own small box on the H administrative chart. In a still higher court, Vice President Nelson Rockefeller had worked successfully, though not without difficulty, toward one of their chief concerns, the creation of a White House office of science, engineering and technology policy, absent since a comparable office had been abolished by President Nixon in 1973.

Cooper had come up with something new, a Forward Plan for Health in which "knowledge development" was a predominant theme; and he seemed to be holding his own against OMB budget trimming. A Presidential panel was listening to NIH concerns. On predominantly Democratic Capitol Hill there was ambivalence; although the majority showed sympathy for the NIH when it suffered at the hands of the administration, it showed impatience too, for concrete achievements.

In Dr. Donald Fredrickson, the NIHers had a self-confident scientist-leader. Fredrickson, a Republican, had been offered his job before Cooper, but had delayed accepting, knowing he must be able to work in tandem with whomever was chosen for the top H job. The Cooper-Fredrickson combination, while not intimate, seemed to be working: the NIH had once again begun to act, not just react, to a barrage of outside demands. One read and heard on the grapevine, not of complaints and resignations, but of activities and initiatives.

Item: Director Fredrickson called a two day meeting during which rules governing the controversial area of genetic research moved closer to reality, a nationally publicized gathering on a hot topic unlikely to have taken place on the NIH campus during the Nixon era. A year and a half earlier, scientists had called for a moratorium on recombinant DNA (deoxyribonucleic acid) research in which the active material of the genes that govern heredity can be transplanted and rearranged. Tampering with nature's reproductive processes can lead to revolutionary improvements in human health or to dangerous unknown perils. At Fredrickson's meeting, scientists and lawyers and others concerned worked over a set of draft guidelines for NIH-sponsored research which would be of great potential influence on other research as well.

Item: The Clinical Center, whose cornerstone was laid by President Harry S. Truman, is badly in need of modernization. This research hospital central to the NIH intramural effort needs at least $14 million worth of repairs (including the updating of an operating room which had fallen far below standard), and since more and more health care takes place outside of hospital beds these days, it needs a new $72 million ambulatory unit. Fredrickson toured Congressmen, HEW and OMB officials through the Center, and, as Assistant Secretary Cooper admitted with some satisfaction, "pushed us pretty hard". The results were good: over $21 million appeared in the President's Fiscal Year 1977 budget to begin the refurbishing job. The Director also brought top Clinical Center staff together at the Tidewater Inn in Maryland to thrash out fundamentals of Clinical Center care policy—matters that, he said, had not been thoroughly discussed for twenty-five years.

High on the list of problems facing Dr. Fredrickson: recruitment. During the Golden Years, the NIH Associate Program had attracted to the Clinical Center young physician researchers of the highest quality. "We were like a medical research Tiffany's" he remembers, "gathering up precious stones." Competition to enter was keen; the intramural program served as a rigorous training ground not only for the NIH leadership but for medical school faculties around the country and so for all American medicine. Now applications have dropped discouragingly. In 1968, a young person applying for admission to the NIH program was one of 755 applicants for about 200 vacancies (all were filled); by 1975 applicants had shrunk to 211 for the same number of vacancies (only 92 were filled). In the same period the applicants for the NHLI program had dropped from 432 (9 were selected) to 112 (the NHLI intramural chief, Dr. Jack Orloff, interviewed less than 80, and 11 were picked).

In a sense, NIH has been a victim of its own success; it must now compete for recruits with other fine medical research centers, often led by its own alumni. Many blame the end of the doctor draft for the drop in applicants, and indeed some young doctors oriented to research chose service at Bethesda in lieu of military service in Viet Nam, or in another era, Korea. But the absence of the doctor draft at the foot of the ladder could be said to resemble the $37,800 ceiling at the top; though it helps discourage people, it would not be as great a drawback if NIH had retained its once lustrous image.

Director Fredrickson, most agreed, had set about polishing up that image. But no one was more aware than this engaging, sometimes imperious scientist administrator of the formidable nature of that job.

One thing was sure: the golden era, the years of unqualified acceptance, had passed for NIH, as for all of medicine. Money was tight—but it was a question of attitudes and priorities as well as money. Few questioned that NIH and health research could no longer take the lion's share of the H or Public Health Service budget; indeed, commentators pointed out that the NIHers had cried wolf too often, over a budget which had doubled since 1968 (although it had increased in real dollars only about 25 percent, and most of that increase had gone to cancer, and to a far lesser extent, heart and lung research.) Few questioned either that NIH also had to compete, in a time of inflation and unprecedented peacetime budget deficits, with enormous open-ended non-H commitments in its own Department, like Medicare and Medicaid, which were paying for health care for more old and poor and sick people.* The big questions concerned the function—or dysfunction—of the whole health care system. How to see that the best health care in Manhattan is available in Keokuk as well? How to contain the costs of such care and still assure its widespread use? How to deliver it in a less fragmented and more rational way?

But oddly, even among the so-called free spenders in Congress, many were persuaded that the federal health dollar had become finite—and few questioned the appropriateness of priorities that placed the NIH health research budget ($1.7 billion of the total $2 billion NIH budget) at about the same figure as the cost of one Trident submarine ($1.65 billion). Even an official like Dr. Cooper, who spends a great deal of time defending the health dollar, told a meeting of prominent biologists at the end of 1975 that HEW's budget is now bigger than the Defense Department's. Perhaps he conceded too much, because the $128 billion HEW budget includes the Social Security and Medicare trust funds which together produced some $90 billion in benefits that year; without these

---

*In 1968, NIH's budget was $1.1 billion, the rest of the Public Health Service's $1.7 billion; by 1975, NIH's budget had grown to $2 billion and the rest of the Public Health Service's to $3.2 billion; Medicare and Medicaid together accounted for some $25 billion in federal dollars.

benefits, previously bought and paid for, HEW's budget shrank to $38 billion as compared to the Defense Department's $91 billion. At an HEW press briefing on the Administration's 1977 budget proposals, no one paid much attention to NIH at all, except to ask why, for the first time in many a year, had no new funds been proposed for cancer research?

So, the struggle for control of the finite federal health dollar and for containment of health costs had become a hallmark of the new era. Another was confusion. A great deal of lip service had been paid to the benefits research produces in preventing disease—in dollars as well as pain. But people tend to forget the great savings when a polio vaccine replaces a lifetime iron lung machine. They may not understand the difficulties involved in attacking chronic diseases which develop over a period of many years, and which may have many causes, not just one. They wonder about charges and counter charges surrounding the efficacy and safety of, for example, a birth control pill. They wonder at the increasing evidence that they can get sick just by living in the environment they had thought sustained them. When Dr. Howard M. Temin, American cancer researcher and long time NIH grantee, walked to the podium to claim his 1975 Nobel Prize for Medicine, he seemed to sum it all up: he told the hushed crowd of royalty and commoners to stop smoking (hundreds, it was reported, crushed out their cigarettes, but lit up again as soon as he finished his short speech). No matter how much science has tried, Temin explained, its work has not led to a cure for cancer, but he was outraged at the lack of measures taken to stop cigarette smoking.

Yet another hallmark of the new era was the subtle shift in attitude toward all things medical, including medical research. Hard questions were being asked that no one would have dreamed of asking a decade ago. What are you doing with our tax dollars and why? Are you working to serve all of us equitably? Are you emphasizing the work most likely to help me and my children ten years from now? Are you taking care

181

that you do not harm the world we leave to future generations? Are you developing a cure for *my* mother's disease? Are you spending money on research you should be spending on health education?

Americans had always been eager for the best available health care, at a cost they could afford, for themselves and for their families. With television bringing the latest medical miracles right into their living rooms, this feeling intensified. Politicians with sensitive antennae were not surprised at a report of a Patrick Caddell poll taken in the summer of 1975: most of the men and women interviewed wanted more government spending for health care. Thirty-five percent wanted some sort of national health insurance which would guarantee them as much health care as they needed; another 22 percent opted for the most extreme solution, a nationalized health system in which, not only would health care be guaranteed, but doctors and hospitals would be taken over by the government, and fees, salaries, and prices regulated.

Within this new ambience, politics representing people wanting, in the words of Tolstoi's hero, Ivan Ilych, "to live and not to suffer", had created a whole complex of pressures surrounding the NIHers as they go about their job. These pressures—some demands, some mere feelings—are difficult to categorize. Each criss-crosses and impinges on the other, some are philosophical, or ideological, some budgetary. Let us divide them, somewhat arbitrarily, into three sets:

1. The first set centers around demands for more NIH accountability. In governmentese, there are two sorts of accountability. The traditional meaning concerns fiscal accounting—knowing where public monies go and assuming proper responsibility for their expenditure. In that respect, NIH has always performed well; most wonder that in thirty years of funding some 254,000 research grants totalling $10.4 billion through the peer review system, the agency has never suffered a serious scandal.

What members of Congress mean when they challenge NIH accountability is something quite different. They are saying that the public, having invested billions of dollars in the Institutes' work, should have obtained a quicker and better return on its investment, and by return they mean effective weapons against the modern chronic killers.

There is another dimension to accountability. The NIH traditionally has positioned itself above the battle, protecting the biomedical scientists, trying to see that they be left to do their research, undistracted. A small but symbolic example: when NIH information men recommended highway signs indicating the location of the NIH campus, their suggestion was ignored. (Holding an open house for the community in conjunction with the 1975 Alumni meeting was a triumph for communications over scientific reticence.) It takes time and patience to conduct a dialogue, and some prima donnas of biomedicine have been above trying to interpret intelligibly for laymen. There is always the danger that reporters will not include all the limitations and qualifications which characterize scientific papers. The result was a hushed silence over the lawns of Bethesda, broken only by occasional pronouncements *ex cathedra*. The downtown policy makers naturally often found NIHers unresponsive or resistant when asked to give an accounting for their work or to increase their efforts in this or that direction.

The post-Golden Years NIH leaders were not strong enough to stave off growing impatience with the NIH progress. Many (including the Laskerites) considered it overly passive to wait for ideas to emanate from grant applications. This impatience took different forms as the years went by. At first, the approach of the policy makers was drastic: a War on Cancer under a revamped, quasi-independent National Cancer Institute which could bypass the NIH director and his HEW superiors in budget, program and personnel matters and structure its own research projects in a number of new ways. The research community's dissatisfaction with this imbalanced

183

cancer program led to a mobilization of biomedical leadership which succeeded in holding the war on heart disease to a lower key. The National Heart and Lung Institute got more money to mount a broader, larger program, but the Institute stayed within NIH and gained no special access to high political power.

Next the Congress made more frequent and formal use of the Disease of the Month Club approach. (Targeting instructions had long been given by appropriation committees; now they were being written into authorization legislation.) A consensus grew that further imbalance and fragmentation among the Institutes were to be avoided. So were new Institutes, which cost more money, carried heavy overhead charges, and might prove counterproductive. Nevertheless, an Institute on Aging was created at the behest of a determined lobby for senior citizens.

Aside from the scientists' view that Congressional or political targets did not necessarily coincide with scientific opportunity, the practical problem here was that extra funding did not always accompany specific targeting; when a constituency was strong, as in the case of the sickle cell target, money was carved out of NHLI to attack it; when it was not, as in the case of Cooley's anemia, the degree of dedication depended on those to whom the target was assigned. Fearing that such targeting could sprout hundreds of separate programs, scientists pointed out that a very large number of ills may be inherited, and successfully urged legislators to work toward an overall approach to genetic diseases.

But the notion of gaining some sort of visibility and special NIH attention for a disease persisted: even the addition of a name to an Institute seemed to reap results. Though purists objected when 15 percent of the NHLI budget was carved out for lung disease, the consensus now is that pulmonary research has benefited from its marriage to the large cardiovascular effort. Now, the advocacy of organized hematologists is adding the word "Blood" to the NHLI title.

Some say that the Commission of the Month has replaced the Disease of the Month Club approach; others that it is simply a horse of a slightly different color. Take the Diabetes Commission, created by the Congress in response to strenuous lobbying on the part of Americans who felt *their* disease was not getting its proper share of attention. This Commission, after intensive study, called for tripling the funds attacking diabetes by 1980 and setting up a super-advisory board at the Assistant Secretary for Health echelon to oversee the research, treatment and education effort. Introducing a bill to make this possible, Pennsylvania's Senator Richard S. Schweiker said this special outside-NIH board was needed because research on diabetes, the country's third most serious health problem, was currently being conducted by seven of the Institutes, and "as we all know, everyone's responsibility is no one's responsibility".

One thing is sure: the Institutes were built on political demands for categorical research in the cause of better health. These demands naturally increase in a time when awareness of many rights, including the right to health care, is growing. The potential power of disease constituencies was illustrated when the President's Biomedical Research Panel considered recommending that each Institute contribute one to two percent of its budget to a flexible central fund which the NIH Director could use for promising new opportunities which might arise between Congressional hearings. Old hands thought this suggestion impossible: the Institutes' constituencies want public monies spent on *their* research demands, not someone else's.

Recently NIH Director Dr. Donald Fredrickson said he understood such demands: "We will go the whole route in trying to satisfy them". But, he added, "you cannot keep running down to the cellar to get the ingredients to bake the cake unless the ingredients are there". As pressure for accountability has grown, so has the responsiveness of the modern generation of NIH leaders. The other side of the coin is

185

the growing awareness, even among advocates of strong disease campaigns, of the truth of Fredrickson's observation: to bake the cake you need the ingredients. (Look, for example, at Cancer Panel Chairman Benno Schmidt's strong advocacy of the necessity for a fundamental science base, or at the fact that almost 70 percent of the Congressionally-targeted Houston Supercenter first year budget goes to its Division of Basic Research.) The trick for the new era will be to balance the growing consensus about the importance of basic research with the demands for accountability, and to do so with intelligence and statesmanship.

2. The second set of pressures confronting NIH concerns the agency's mission. Outgoing NIH Director Dr. Robert Stone told his last Advisory Committee meeting that the question of this mission had been the source of more pain to him than any other. Well, what should it be? What activities should NIH pursue; what role should it assume?

During the 1950s and early 1960s, the National Institutes of Health clearly enjoyed a single, prestigious, non-controversial role: it was a research agency, dedicated to the development of knowledge, where microbe hunters and doctor-investigators bent over their test tubes and their patients in the pursuit of truth. Today, the Institutes are asked not only to seek basic knowledge through research and then clinical trials, but to demonstrate how that knowledge can control disease, and how to educate both medical professionals and the public in its use.

As we have seen in our look at the National Heart and Lung Institute program, and at the Houston Supercenter, the largest piece of the budget pie is still going to the individual investigators. But the Institutes are being pushed along the research delivery continuum and the scientists are being joined by all sorts of co-workers never there before, from communications specialists to ambulance teams.

This has happened as the feeling has grown that somehow the nation has not exploited the knowledge that we have. We

186

know smoking causes lung cancer and helps bring on heart disease—how can we persuade young people not to start what may become a pleasurable habit? We know how to control high blood pressure—how can we cajole independently minded Americans into effective treatment? The economists tell us we could save great amounts of money by answering such questions and public health oriented physicians say we could lengthen lives*—it only takes common sense to see that an ounce of prevention is worth a pound of cure.

Interestingly enough, the Congress has turned to NIH to find answers to such questions, not because the agency has been doing a bad job, but because it has done a good one. Other health agencies, most logically the Health Services Administration and the Center for Disease Control, could pick up where NIH leaves off to demonstrate and educate. But there is no other agency with the same prestige, and with access to the best and brightest medical stars, in this country and abroad.

Some say that NIH has played the reluctant dragon when asked to take on unfamiliar new assignments. Indeed, it is true that many have held back, explaining that they have neither the community public health skills nor experience required. They

---

*An extreme example: A study done in Alameda County, California by distinguished public health authority Dr. Lester Breslow and statistician Nedra B. Belloc showed that if you follow seven old-fashioned simple rules, your chances of enjoying good health and longer life would increase: 1. Don't smoke cigarettes. 2. If you drink alcohol, do so in moderation. 3. Eat breakfast. 4. Don't eat between meals. 5. Maintain normal weight. 6. Sleep seven or eight hours a day. 7. Exercise moderately. There is little medical quarrel with rules one and two. But some doctors point out that admonitions about hygienic living (though tempting to policymakers because advice is cheap) may not apply in individual cases, where a host of factors, including heredity and environment, play significant parts. Also a self selection process reduces the significance of the rules. They are likely to be observed best by people who are healthy.

187

have another point: service-oriented programs have a way of eating into basic research budgets. Whenever you start treating patients, whether research jargon terms your program "demonstration" or "control" or something else, you run smack into the twin problems of human health needs and spiralling medical costs. The National Heart and Lung Institute has taken on about $15 million in demonstration and education programs aimed to show how better to control disease—mostly in hypertension and sickle cell disease. Since no extra monies have been appropriated for such work nor for the big clinical trials, now costing the Institute $40-60 million, such programs are squeezing individually-initated research.

On the other hand, Congress not only mandated the Cancer Institute's control programs, but appropriated funds for them. These programs, covering whole communities, seek to demonstrate that by intervening in every possible way, say in breast or lung cancer care of specific populations, you can decrease the cancer toll. The expectation is that local communities, which share in the costs (now well over $50 million*) will pick up the total tab when their federal support runs out. Officials worry that this expectation may never be fulfilled.

The mental health experience has sounded a warning, too. The expert consensus is that research in this area suffered in both quantity and quality when it was combined in one organization with services. This happened first at the National Institute of Mental Health, and later at the Alcohol, Drug and Mental Health Administration (ADAMHA),—the three-institute sister organization of NIH created in 1973. Alcoholism, drug abuse, and mental illness are urgent national problems, and this is a time of great promise for the study of the brain and its serious and subtle effects on the human body. Yet the President's Biomedical Research Panel found that ADAMHA's service responsibilities leave it too little capabili-

---

*The budget of the entire Eye Institute is some $44 million, and of Environmental Health, $34 million.

ty to conduct vigorously this urgently needed research. (The NIMH probably is the best off of the three ADAMHA Institutes, and the NIMH intramural program which remains on the NIH campus is considered excellent).

When a group of 26 prominent Americans, including Mary Lasker, Dr. Jonas Salk and Margaret Mead, telegraphed the Panel asking that it consider the creation of a new Population Institute, it turned the idea aside after brief consideration, and recommended merely beefing up research on reproductive biology through existing structures. Not only was it wary of the difficulties involved in creating new institutes, but it did not want to run the risk of bringing the family planning service programs administered in other parts of the Public Health Service or H into NIH.

The complex question of NIH's mission is baffling, but not insoluble. Clearly, the raw ore of research must be refined before it can be used. One scenario for accomplishing the refinement job reads something like this: let NIH continue with its basic and clinical research work and supervise the clinical trials which follow (but be sure trials are separately budgeted). Let NIH also conduct small, time-limited carefully evaluated demonstration or control programs (as the NHLI is doing at the Houston Supercenter) on how this knowledge can best be used. Let it work out ways to disseminate this knowledge both to medical practitioners, and to the public (as is increasingly necessary when people must take more responsibility for their own health).

Then draw the line. Let other agencies manage large scale demonstration or control programs—perhaps the Health Services Administration, perhaps the Center for Disease Control with its widespread contacts in state health departments. Make sure that clear methods are worked out whereby NIH can advise and consult with other agencies, on a reimbursable basis, reviewing, appraising and monitoring the validity and cost of knowledge applications.

Policy makers are groping toward such a scenario, for, as NIH Director Fredrickson puts it, "There is something too informal about the collegial system for validations of applications and something too haphazard about the methods for their distribution and continuing appraisal." If the country adopts some sort of a system of national health insurance before roles and missions are agreed on, the NIH could be snowed under by demands for guidance. The government would need to turn to some knowledgeable health agency for assurance that it is getting the effective health care it is paying for. If that agency turned out to be NIH alone, presumably because it was still the only organization with prestige enough to do the job, the Institutes would have time and resources for little else.

3. This brings us to the third set of issues or pressures which for lack of a better word, we can call psychological. How do NIHers feel about their work? How do they perceive their agency? How do they feel about biomedical research? How do their peers feel about them? Do bright young people considering research careers look to them as models? Do they want to become senior or principal investigators at the Clinical Center or outside, in NIH funded projects in medical academe?

To some, as one eminent biomedical scientist put it, the "extraordinary esthetic experience that is science" is "the only way". For them the excitement of the search for understanding about man and his relation to the earth—if they are free to conduct that search within reasonable bounds—transcends outside annoyances and prerequisites. They are ready to get on with the job. For others, especially among the older NIHers who are extraordinarily attached to their institution and its tradition of excellence, the past five years have seemed lean and difficult. To repeat one senior NHLI physician-administrator: "When I came here as a young man, my friends thought I was coming to the Taj Mahal. Now they would ask, 'What the hell for? Not for the money!' "

Many factors contribute to such a feeling; some very real, some blown out of proportion: NIH's shabby treatment during the early Nixon era; the War on Cancer and Disease of the

190

Month Club approaches; the as yet unclear role of the NIH within the federal government; the fear that biomedical scientists do not have enough say in health research decision-making; the feeling of some researchers, especially clinical investigators, that they are hemmed in by contemporary consumer and patient rights rules, regulations and guidelines.

To young people attracted to medical research, some of these issues may seem dated. A prevailing worry for them is instability. They are naturally wary of a future where their role and independence is unclear. More immediately, they are wary of an off-again, on-again system which promises opportunities one day, and reneges the next. Especially for the young M.D.s, as one put it, there is too much money in medical practice and too much hassle in research. Suggestions for antidotes like funding biomedical research at a steady rate—say an annual level which would maintain real growth at between 4 and 5 percent—are not usually pleasing to members of Congress. They want the final say as to how and where public health monies are spent.

To be fair, one must note again that the NIHers have not been especially adept at communicating their hopes and fears, not only to their lords and masters in the Administration and Congress, but to the public. Many officials have found them unable or unwilling to answer questions, and have accused them of scientific arrogance or a "just give us the money and let us spend it" attitude. This does not sit well in an era where public questioning is the rule. When they resisted a demand under the Freedom of Information Act to disclose details of grants which NIMH had awarded, they had a reason: applicants could be reluctant to describe the design of their experiments if they knew competitors might take their ideas and run with them. (Dr. James D. Watson, the Nobelist and co-discoverer of the structure of DNA, has described the intense competitiveness of high science in *The Double Helix.**)

---

*The Double Helix: A Personal Account of the Discovery of the Structure of DNA. Atheneum, 1968.

But The District of Columbia Court of Appeals compelled disclosure and asked whether NIH did not consider the biomedical scientists "a meanspirited lot who pursue self-interest as ruthlessly as the Barbary pirates in their own chosen field".

The difficulty the scientists have in communicating their views was epitomized in a naive press conference held by the Federation of American Scientists at the time of Dr. Robert Stone's dismissal as NIH director. The organization produced the three Nobelists at NIH as well as other distinguished NIH biomedical men to deplore his dismissal and the politicization of NIH research.

Those were, as Mr. Rogers calls them, the difficult days. Morale was at low ebb. Malaise prevailed; the Institutes were leaderless, unrepresented. Even at the NHLI, comparatively favored as we have seen, worthwhile grant applications increasingly remained unfunded, monies had to be diverted from basic research to support a public education program, Disease of the Month Club research and clinical trials were squeezing basic research, training programs were in an uproar and prospective trainees turned off. If that were true at Heart, surely even more disquieting examples could have been found at the smaller Institutes. Still, the glamorous FAS panel members could not satisfy the reporters who wanted to know why they were unhappy with a $2 billion budget. Nor could they make the former Director into a martyr. "We want our scientists at NIH left, as much as possible, alone to do their thing", the FAS statement read. It sounded not only petulant, but self-serving. (Dr. Nirenberg, articulate in a one-to-one interview, said nothing at the press conference.)

Looking at these pressures in those same difficult days, the NHLI's Dr. W. French Anderson observed that they were "like waves which have not gotten here yet, but which are getting closer". What worried him and his investigator colleagues was that, if the waves did engulf NIH, it could not survive as a place of excellence. With the Golden Years gone, political figures unfamiliar with the biomedical scientists' work and ignorant of its long range value might be able to tell them to study this, or study that, though it made no scientific sense and was done for other than health research reasons. Then they would become slaves to the politician's love of the limelight, or the administrator's preoccupation with cost-effectiveness, or the well-intentioned layman's idea of what disease should be cured tomorrow. NIH would become a Bureau of Dogs and Cats, a place for old hands and second rate scientists, where everyone arrives and leaves on time, and everything is reported in memos written in perfect bureaucratese, and reflected in impressive cost-effectiveness charts, but where the public good is not served, for little knowledge is gained and no preventives or cures produced.

But that has not happened. The waves have not engulfed NIH—yet. A Presidential Panel on Biomedical Research financed by $2.5 million of NIH money has studied them in detail. This Congressionally mandated panel had a difficult time producing constructive recommendations in an uncertain Presidential election year. As the hearings closed, it seemed unlikely that the panel would rock the boat. Its report would, however, strongly support the work of NIH and its less fortunate sister, ADAMHA, and suggest various ways of bolstering them, including the establishment of a series of Presidentially appointed advisory boards and panels which could give the whole research system greater access to the political ear. Then various Congressional committees would begin oversight hearings to air the panel's recommendations.

The panel did not recommend that the dominance and special privileges of the Cancer Institute be tampered with; Benno Schmidt had made sure of that. But it did propose that the President's Cancer Panel with its special status take over as President's Panel for all biomedical research. Some felt this suggestion opened the door a notch to the eventual restoration of balance between the institutes; others that it would give the Cancer Panel and its politically savvy, pro-cancer Chairman Schmidt still greater authority. What will come out of all this

193

remains an unanswered question. Clearly the politics of health research is entering a new era—an era in which many more people are involved and the complexities of meeting human health needs have multiplied enormously.

The pressures on the NIH as it goes about its research job—Dr. French Anderson's oncoming waves—will not abate. Elected officials will continue to want to have a say in the public's $2 billion annual investment in health research. The Congress has reformed its budget process and showed it wants to set its own priorities. Legislative self assertiveness, intensified during the prolonged confrontation with President Nixon, takes many forms. One is a trend toward limited, rather than open-ended, authorization acts. At present it has reached only the Cancer and Heart Institutes, but it could provide another lever for Congressional power over all the institutes.

Still, the pressures can turn into opportunities as well as problems. The common sense of the people, as reflected in their representatives, is, taken collectively, as good a rudder for government as has been discovered thus far. Having invested as much as it has in the National Institutes of Health, elected officials will probably find that it only makes sense to try to maintain the agency as a center of excellence, a place respected throughout the world for its preeminent contributions to medicine.

Continued preeminence will require a great deal from many different people. Those we have called the NIHers—at NIH itself and in the biomedical community across the country—will need to balance their step by step progress from one discovery to the next with a flexible response to public needs and aspirations. Recognizing that they are part of the larger society, they will have to display a willingness to try new ways, to lend their expertise, and, importantly, to help the public understand what they have done, what they are doing, and what they want to do. Recognizing the limitations of biomedical science, all of us, and those who represent us in government, will have to confine our demands to what is reasonable and achievable within the contemporary state of the art.

Asked by Senate Health Appropriations Subcommittee Chairman Magnuson in early 1976 whether the past few years' trend toward decreased deaths from heart attacks was continuing, NHLI Director Robert Levy was able to answer "yes".

He reported that heart attack rates had dropped over nine percent in the five years between 1968 and 1973, and three percent more between 1973 and 1975. No single new effective or therapeutic measure had been applied to the whole population and could be credited with the change. Many factors seemed to be involved, including improved control of hypertension or high blood pressure which is associated with heart attacks, a decrease in the number of men over 35 who smoke cigarettes, and an explosive increase in our ability to diagnose and treat coronary artery disease.

Statistics like these are the Institutes' best bulwark against the oncoming waves. If such progress can continue, and can be made against other ills as well, perhaps one day we can all look forward to a happy and healthy life, like the Deacon's Masterpiece—that "wonderful one-hoss shay, that was built in such a logical way it ran a hundred years to a day and went to pieces all at once, and nothing first, just as bubbles do when they burst."

Index

197

Caddell, Patrick poll, 182
Cancer Act of 1971, 41-4, 74
Cardiac Replacement (Ad Hoc Task Force Report), 158-60, 166
Center for Disease Control, 187, 189
Clinical Center (of NIH), 8, 12, 15, 24, 30, 69-71, 84, fn. 128, 154, 159, 178-9, 190
Cohen, Wilbur J., 13, 16, 128
Committee of Consultants on Cancer, 40-1, 53-4
Comroe, Dr. Julius H., Jr., 37, 47, 170
Congressional Black Caucus, 80, 87
Congressional Budget and Impoundment Control Act of 1974, 118
Congressional Research Service, 129
Conlan, Rep. John, 47
Cooley, Dr. Denton A., 144, 155-7
Cooper, Dr. John A.D., 130
Cooper, Dr. Theodore, 8, 9, 21, 33, 53-4, 57, 156, 162, 166, 173, 177-8, 180
Coulson, Dr. Richard, 95-6, 110
Cranston, Sen. Alan, 89-90, 97
Crick, Sir Francis, 72
Culliton, Barbara J., fn. 50

DeBakey, Dr. Michael E., 3, 28, 51-2, 55-6, 59-62, 67-8, 103, 108, 145, 150, 152, 155-6
Department of Defense (DOD), 15, 145, 180
Deykin, Dr. Daniel, 94, 110
Dirks, Harley, 119
Division of Research Grants (NIH) 20, 43, 46
Downey, Herman, fn. 128
Dripps, Dr. Robert D., 37
Dryden, Hugh, 145
DuVal, Dr. Merlin K., 129

Dyer, Dr. Rolla, 23
Ebert, Dr. Robert H., 125
Edwards, Dr. Charles C., 127, 177
Ehrlichman, John, 14, 78
Eisenhower, President Dwight D., 24
Energy Research and Development Administration (ERDA—formerly part of AEC), 151, 167
Estabrook, Dr. Ronald W., 135-6
Evans, Dr. Richard I., 64, 67

Farber, Dr. Sidney, 29
Farrell, Sylvia, 52
Federation of American Scientists, 17, 192
Federation of American Societies for Experimental Biology, 136
Flood, Rep. Daniel J., 172
Fogarty, Rep. John E., 25, 27-8, 34, 36, 142-3, 145-7, 172
Folsom, Marion, 28
Food, Drug and Cosmetics Act of 1962, 159
Ford, President Gerald, 20, 41, 49, 71; Administration, 6, 9, 17
Fountain, Rep. Lawrence H., 32
Fox, Renée C., 154, fn. 157
Framingham, Mass. heart studies, 30, 104
Fredrickson, Dr. Donald S., 7-9, 21-2, 61, 147, 149, 153, fn. 159, 173, 177-9, 185-6
Friedman, Dr. Ephraim, 127
Frommer, Dr. Peter, 154, 166

Gardner, John, 28, 32, 72
General Accounting Office, 18, 129
Georgetown University Medical Center, 135
Giaimo, Rep. Robert N., 80-2
Glazer, Shep, 161

198

Glenn, John, 52
Goldman, LeRoy, 76
Gorman, Mike, 26, 55, 57, 71
Gotto, Dr. Antonio M., Jr., 61-2, 66
Grasso, Gov. Ella T. (former Representative), 75, 80, 82
Green, Dr. Jerome, 53
Green, Harold P., 162
Grondin, Dr. Pierre, 155
Guiliotis, Dorothy, 80-3
Guyton, Dr. Arthur C., 136
"H", colloquialism for the six Public Health Service agencies, 9, 14, 56, 189
Haldeman, H. Robert, 14
Harmison, Dr. Lowell T., 150, 152, fn. 162
Harris, Sen. Fred, 160
Hart, Sen. Gary, 169
Harvard University, 8, 28, 42, 97, 123, 125
Harvey, Dr. Proctor, 135
Hastings Center Reports of the Institute of Society, Ethics and the Life Sciences, fn. 163
Hastings, Dr. Frank, 145, 147, 150, 166
Health and the Environment (formerly Public Health and Environment) Subcommittee of the House Interstate and Foreign Commerce Committee, 18, 19, 120-123, 132, 172
Health Services Administration, 187, 189
Health Subcommittee of the Senate Labor and Public Welfare Committee, 8, 25, 127-132, 170
Heart attacks, 24, 30-3, 103-6, 136, 148, 195
Heart transplants, 153-160
Hill, Sen. Lister, 25, 27, 33, 36, fn. 128, 171

Horning, Prof. Evan, 65, 67
Horowitz, Dr. Lawrence, 130
Howard University, 79
Hypertension, 63, 66, 87, 108
Hygienic Laboratory (became NIH), 22, 74
Iglehart, John K., 128
Insull, Dr. William, Jr., 94-5, 110
Iovene, Michael, 80-2
Jackson, Dr. Rudolph, 88
Jasper, Herbert, 161
Javits, Sen. Jacob, 40, 41, 50
Johnson, President Lyndon B., 13, 32-3, 52, 55
Johnson, Robert Wood Foundation, 129
Jonsen, Dr. Albert R., fn. 163, 165
Kantrowitz, Dr. Adrian, 152
Kaplan, Dr. Henry S., 43
Kaplan, Morris Bernard, fn. 163
Karp, Mr. & Mrs. Haskell, 155-7
Kelly, James, 16
Kennedy, Sen. Edward M., 8, 16, 17, 41-2, 50, 82, 90, 127, 130-3, 169, 171
Kennedy, President John F., 27
Kennedy, Dr. Thomas J., 120
King, Colbert, 78, 79
Kirschstein, Dr. Ruth, fn. 99
Klitgaard, Dr. Howard M., 114
Knutti, Dr. Ralph E., 142-8
Kolff, Dr. Willem J., 144-5, 152
Kornberg, Dr. Arthur, 9-10, 29, 160
Lambis, Judy, 69-72, 82-3
Lambis, Nick, 69-72, 82-3
Landers, Ann, 42
Lasker, Mary, 16, 26-8, 32-3, 36, 56, 71, 173-4, 189; Lasker forces or lobby, 27, 28, 32, 39, 40, 43, 183
Lawton, Stephan, 130
Lederberg, Dr. Joshua, 43, 143
Levine, Dr. Peter H., 96-7, 110

202